The Childless Marriage –
An Exploratory Study of Couples Who Do Not Want Children

The Childless Marriage

*An Exploratory Study of Couples
Who Do Not Want Children*

D
6.5
CAM

Elaine Campbell

Tavistock Publications
London and New York

First published in 1985 by
Tavistock Publications Ltd
11 New Fetter Lane, London EC4P 4EE

Published in the USA by
Tavistock Publications
in association with Methuen, Inc.
29 West 35th Street, New York, NY 10001

Photoset by
Nene Phototypesetters Ltd, Northampton
Printed in Great Britain
by Richard Clay (The Chaucer Press) Ltd,
Bungay, Suffolk

British Library Cataloguing in Publication Data
Campbell, Elaine
The childless marriage: an exploratory study
of couples who do not want children.
1. Childlessness – Social aspects – Scotland
I. Title
304.6'66   HQ766.5.G7

ISBN 0–422–60060–1
ISBN 0–422–60070–9 Pbk

Library of Congress Cataloging in Publication Data
Campbell, Elaine.
The childless marriage.
Bibliography: p.
Includes indexes.
1. Childlessness – Scotland – Case studies.
2. Married people – Scotland – Case studies.
3. Choice (Psychology)   I. Title.
HQ618.C36   1985   306.8'5   85–14705

ISBN 0–422–60060–1
ISBN 0–422–60070–9 (pbk.)

To my children, Victoria and Andrew,
I hope you think your sacrifices were worthwhile

Contents

Preface

On March 20, 1984, in response to an article by Jane McLoughlin, 'The case for the conscientious objector to motherhood', a woman wrote to *The Guardian*, 'It is surely time to bring this debate (on the ethics of married women opting out of motherhood) into the open, to let all those disbelieving mums know there are in fact married women who have other aims in life, to make confidently expectant would-be grandparents accept that they may have to face disappointment'. There followed further correspondence. Fran Bagenal, for example, noted how 'revealing' it was 'that the three letters full of the joys of motherhood were signed while the woman "lacking the maternal urge" felt the need to remain anonymous' (March 27). In the early 1970s, the feminist Shulamith Firestone made a similar observation, fearing physical violence against women who shed their anonymity (Firestone 1972). Voluntary child-lessness is an emotive issue. On the one hand, the con-servative sees it as further evidence of the self-indulgence that is tearing the nuclear family apart and threatening the fabric of society; whilst on the other, the radical applauds it as demonstration of the increasing role of individualism and democracy in the intimate relations between men, women, and children, and as a means for greater self-fulfilment. This book set out neither to condemn nor to justify the men and women who took this decision, but to give them a long overdue opportunity to speak for themselves – to air the views *The Guardian's* correspondent believed should be aired. Those offered the opportunity took it willingly, often frankly thankful to be able to 'bring the debate into the open', to be able confidently to shed their anonymity.

I had rejected as simplistic prevailing explanations of their behaviour as pathological or indicative of inadequacy; these seemed to me to ignore totally the ability men and women have to bend the rules, to side-step dominant values and norms when they so desire. I wanted to know how couples became childless, how the desire emerged and was translated into action; my interest was in situations and motives and not in the structural conditions so many sociologists of fertility had seen as determining reproductive behaviour. Mine was a humanistic approach in a field of study that until recently had been dominated by the assumptions of positivist sociology.

I could not have pursued this aim without the cooperation of the women and men who are the subjects of this study. They generously shared their perceptions, emotions, and experiences and gave freely of their time and hospitality. Thank you all. Actually finding contacts had been one of my initial worries, but with the help of Dr Nancy Loudon and Dr Margaret Oliver I overcame this problem; to these enthusiastic women I am deeply indebted. I must also mention Arthur Brittan, without whose timely words of encouragement this book would have long since been gathering cobwebs. Thanks are also due to Rosemary Cargill and Helen Wisener who typed the manuscript so proficiently.

Finally, there is Colin Campbell, who has had to live through the difficult times.

1

Childlessness in context

'Thus has been evolved the social type of the "womanly woman", "the normal woman", the chief criterion of normality being a willingness to engage enthusiastically in maternal and allied activities . . . let me quote the following which appeared in a New York newspaper on November 29, 1915: "Only abnormal women want no babies . . . Any woman who does not desire offspring is abnormal".'   (Hollingworth 1916: 22)

'At the present time, for a woman to come out openly against motherhood on principle is physically dangerous. She can get away with it only if she adds that she is neurotic, abnormal, child-hating, and therefore "unfit".'   (Firestone 1972: 189–90)

'It's been a trying year. I was 27 in January, a birthday that's brought on a succession of wheedling phone calls, cosy chats, cornerings in kitchens and outright nagging sessions. The world's decided it's Time Sarah Had A Baby . . . The judgement has been made: despite whatever else I'm doing in my life, I am incomplete, an unfinished woman. And however much I protest my lack of interest in children, it only shows how much I need to be biologically *sorted out* by pregnancy.'
                                                        (Mower 1984)

In 1984, as in 1915, a woman who chooses to remain childless is likely to be censured; she is abnormal, selfish, immature, and possibly neurotic (Busfield and Paddon 1977; Polit 1978; Blake

1979). A man will similarly find himself 'to some degree anomalous and deviant' (Mead 1962: 212). By remaining childless, both sexes are flaunting the basic assumption upon which conventional family life appears to be founded: that once married, all 'healthy', 'normal' adults are committed to accepting, eagerly await, and are well equipped for the parental role (Payne 1978). This is a public image of parenthood epitomized by the young married couple, happy and contented, with toddler on hand and babe in arms. Take the children away and there is no family (Owens 1982). This familiar and simple grouping of parents and offspring embodies a more detailed imagery that provides not only a concise and unambiguous interpretation of what it means to be a parent, but also a motivation to explain and inform reproductive behaviour. In this latter aim it has arguably proved so successful that few question the inevitability of the family round: 'boys are to take over from fathers, girls are to want to produce babies' (Mitchell 1974: 408). Becoming a parent is a foregone conclusion, another example of the taken-for-granted, routine activity that constitutes much of social life (Leibenstein 1981). Reproduction becomes a question of conformity to prevailing values: 'individuals and families living in advanced societies are more and more acting (consciously and unconsciously) under the influence of the cultural values of the society in which they live' (Andorka 1978: 381). This is more an expression of faith on Andorka's part than verified statement since the nature and scope of prevailing norms and values have been given scant consideration (Busfield 1974; Owens 1982). Sociologists as well as demographers have until recently tended to take for granted the inevitability and desirability of parenthood. This dependence upon common sense may have been justified, but was rarely confirmed by empirical findings (a notable exception being Rainwater 1965). The recent upsurge of British and American academic interest in the culture of reproduction does, however, offer some support to this belief in a pervasive pro-natalism (Busfield and Paddon 1977; Payne 1978; Owens 1982; Blake 1979).

Parenthood: the cultural framework

Parenthood remains a valued status, the legitimate goal of most married couples. Peel and Carr (1975) in a study in England and Wales report that only 4 per cent of married couples interviewed admitted they preferred to remain childless. Observation would suggest that both prescriptively and statistically the small family is the norm. In the public image, marriage, parenthood, and the family are inextricably linked; prescribed avenues for those wishing to join the mature, the secure, the respectable, and the adult (Berger and Kellner 1970). Parenthood looms inevitable, but as a key to the adult world of duties and responsibilities it has its compensations: promises of status and approval but also of fun, happiness, love, and affection. Emphasized is the naturalness of parenthood and the harmony of interests between parents, children, and society (Skolnick 1978). Women in particular tend to accept the naturalness, the elementary nature of their desire for offspring, doubting their normality when the maternal urge eludes them and experiencing despair when unable to conceive. Thus the 'ancient value of motherhood' persists (Firestone 1972). There may not be a maternal instinct, in the strict biological sense, and Silverman and Silverman may be justified in their opinion that: 'The greatest pressure that forces women into accepting motherhood was a learned drive that they internalized almost from birth. It was the need to prove their womanhood by having children. It was the Myth of the Maternal Instinct' (1971: 7); but mythical status in no way renders less potent the role of maternal instinct as cultural symbol. If women, and men, believe motherhood to be part of woman's species being then the woman who rejects her anatomical destiny will be perceived as abnormal, unnatural, and incomplete; her mate as abrogating his responsibilities, condoning her abnormality.

For women, parenthood is the natural expression of their femininity, for men, it is a duty to perform. It is a normal activity, to be positively desired, and attained and greeted with joy. Inevitability, naturalness, normality, duty, and romance create what might be characterized as the official interpretation of parental reality: a cultural backcloth to reproductive decisions heavily skewed in favour of the parental role. But whether all social groups share this imagery and accept its unassailable position are questions yet to be adequately answered (MacIntyre 1977; Owens 1982). One thing, however, is certain, and that is that reproductive behaviour has changed and the possibility cannot be ruled out that these changes herald a profound and lasting reorientation of the cultural framework towards greater but not total freedom of reproductive choice. It seems likely that some restrictions on family size will remain; men and women may still be censured for having 'too many' children (Ryder, 1979).

Parenthood: status in retreat?

Since the mid-1960s family-building patterns have changed dramatically throughout the Western world. 'The pattern of the early family with two children has begun to change in every component: there is a larger number of families with no children or an only child, longer intervals between successive births, later age at marriage and a reduction in its frequency, more illegitimate births and more divorces' (OECD 1979: 47). These patterns are translated at the national level into low birth rates (Tabah 1980), so low that in a number of cases the possibility of population decline is fast becoming reality. Whether the trend towards fewer births continues will depend mainly upon the motives that inform couples' reluctance to bear children in numbers sufficient for replacement. The most obvious motive would seem to be economic, since 'fertility tends to decline in periods of depression' (Andorka 1978: 378); an upturn in the economy may therefore be expected to have some stimulating effect upon fertility performance and go some way towards reversing the downward trend in population – as appears to have been the case following the economic depression of the 1930s (Ryder 1979). Reproductive values in this case remain intact, nonconformity being justified in terms of prevailing adverse conditions. Reproductive behaviour, however, is not a simple reflection of economic climate. The relationship is complex and only partially understood. Children are not 'consumer durables' (Blake 1968) and, although economic considerations can and do influence the timing and spacing of births, they determine neither the decision to parent nor ultimate family size (Freedman and Thornton 1982). The economically rational decision would be to have no children (Caldwell 1976). Financial costs, however, do not deter the majority of men and women from marrying and becoming parents. Rather than attempting to maximize utility, they are, Andorka and others suggest, doing what is normal, and what is normal is defined by the cultural framework of values, norms, and images that in all societies attempts to control reproductive activity (Mead 1962). But an increasing number are not doing what is normal unless notions of normality have changed to encompass greater freedom of reproductive choice. Certainly, the technology now exists to allow women to intervene effectively in stages of the reproductive life-cycle they once took for granted, such as menstruation, the menopause, and pregnancy itself.

Unfortunately the relationship between the situations individuals face and emergent reproductive values remains uncharted territory. Whether the availability of effective contraception and the more widespread recourse to legal abortion have produced a situation that negates the call for universal participation by married couples in the reproductive process is open for debate. It can be argued that women have greater control over their bodies than ever before, but the fact that the theoretical possibility exists does not mean that women will use the opportunity it provides to redefine themselves in relation to motherhood. Perhaps the greater threat to pronatalism comes not from technological innovation and its liberating properties but from the increasing demands women are making for equal access to worlds outside the home. Many women work and even more would like to work if they could find adequate care for their children (Oakley 1982); work in itself may not threaten the primacy of the maternal role and may even provide the material opportunity for larger families (Andorka 1978). But women who wish to pursue careers appear to face considerable strategic and emotional difficulties in combining what have been described as the 'incompatible' roles (Komarovsky 1953) of wife-mother/career-woman (Cooper and Davidson 1982). For these women, remaining unmarried or becoming voluntarily childless within marriage may be the 'ultimate liberation' (Movius 1976). Few women make this choice: being wife and mother appears to take precedence over other roles. Nevertheless the existence of alternative life-styles and futures – however remote and strenuous to attain – provides goals the realization of which may require more men and women to question prevailing norms and values, to recognize the possibility of renouncing conventional feminine and masculine aspirations and to formulate their own reproductive careers. Sarah Mower again:

> 'Nice middle-class 70s-educated girls like me were born to equality, scrupulously treated to the same lessons, chores, expectations as our brothers. We were "too good" to learn silly subjects like needlework, cookery, and childcare. Instead we were taught to use our minds, to make decisions based on logic, not emotion. We laughed at this word "feminine" and considered our opportunities to be endless.
>
> Most importantly, I was brought up to independence, to see my life as my own business. I consider I have 10 years in which to think about whether I want children and I'm indignant at suddenly being pushed to obey other people's ideas about "natural female instincts".' (1984)

Analysis and proposed redefinition of the gender roles have of necessity included consideration of the context for which they have the most immediate relevance: the family. While the public image still proclaims the conventional unit of husband, wife, and children as ideal, reality may fall far short of this (Rapoport, Fogarty, and Rapoport 1982). The growing diversity of intimate relationships demands greater tolerance for the unconventional and raises the question of viable alternatives to the nuclear unit. Such critical appreciation extends beyond academic debate into the popular press and media; in the constant quest for a surer path to personal fulfilment, women's magazines in particular have given extensive coverage to the benefits and drawbacks of living outside as well as inside the conventional family. No longer is it taken for granted that individuals always slip neatly and harmoniously into marital and parental roles; it may be natural to marry and have children but to be successful in these roles may require education and guidance. The giving and receiving of personal advice has become a growth industry; specialist magazines – on getting married, having children, remaining single, being a career woman – and television programmes – probing the depths of sexual and familial relationships – proliferate. The assumption is that we can learn to be good lovers, partners, husbands and wives, mothers and fathers.

Being married or a parent is not enough; we now have to measure our success in terms of personal fulfilment and happiness. Those who are not happy or who betray the ideal are no longer automatically judged as abnormal, inadequate, or unfit but in need of expert advice and assistance; only in exceptional cases is it suggested they should be precluded altogether from family life. Family life remains a basic human right, a desirable goal, but is it any longer the only alternative for the 'normal', 'healthy' adult in search of happiness? The search for fulfilment in human relationships does not allow for universals and this search appears to move inexorably forwards, sweeping before it notions of familial duty and obligation (Scanzoni 1983). Marriage is no longer forever nor characterized by mute self-sacrifice but by a more conditional commitment and a degree of self-indulgence. Parenthood's public image has already accommodated promises of joy and happiness to counterbalance notions of duty and obligation, but growing recognition of the difficulties and costs of parenting suggests that those promises are not always realized. Why then conform? Once this question has been asked, routine behaviour becomes active decision making (Leibenstein 1981). Men and women will ask: 'Do *I* have to? What will *I* gain?', or where a joint self-sacrifice is negotiated, 'Do *we* have to? What will *we* gain?' (Yankelovich 1981).

Parenthood appears vulnerable. Not only economic depression and related structural conditions but also conflicting imagery and alternative values and goals provide situations which may facilitate the taking of reproductive decisions that reject the inevitability and desirability of the parental role. One such decision is to marry and remain childless; this is not a popular option. In Britain in the early 70s, when this study began, the number who had actually taken the decision was unknown; a rough estimate using Veevers's method (1972) and the 1971 Census data for Scotland suggests that out of almost a million married women, married once only and at ages under 45, fewer than 2 per cent, or just under 15,000, were childless by choice. Over the previous 20 years the proportions of infertile had in fact declined for women marrying during what appeared to be the most eligible period for subsequent reproduction, the early to mid-20s. Of women aged 45 to 49, effectively those with completed fertility, 7 per cent of those who had married at 20 to

24 and 15 per cent who had married at 25 to 29 were recorded as infertile in 1951, and of these, possibly 2 per cent and 6 per cent respectively were voluntarily childless: by 1961 the proportions of infertile had fallen to 6 per cent and 12 per cent, those voluntarily so down to 1 per cent and 3 per cent; in 1971 the situation remained unchanged. More recent indications are of an increase; how dramatic, however, remains to be seen (Farid 1974; OECD 1979). Prior to the 1970s voluntary childlessness was a 'neglected' area of study (Veevers 1973); according to Veevers this 'neglect . . . reflects to a large extent the value preferences and biases of the social scientists involved . . . they choose to focus the most extensive research on those questions which are congruent with the dominant norms, and, which are supportive of their own preferences' (1973: 199). It might be similarly argued that the upsurge of interest amongst those same social scientists reflects a growing ambiguity in the dominant norms and a widespread questioning of the more basic assumptions of family life. It is also the case that social scientists study 'things which disturb them . . . and those which are experienced as merely puzzling' (Cohen 1976: 9–10); voluntary childlessness fits either category: 'disturbing' those who see it as a growing phe-nomenon threatening population decline, and 'puzzling' those who wish to understand how couples come to reject parenthood in a generally pro-natalist climate. The initial motive-force behind this study contained elements of both positions. Admit-tedly, there was also a more personal note to the investigation: curiosity. Who were the voluntarily childless? How did they make their decision? What pressures did they face and how did they respond? What type of relationships and life-styles did they enjoy? How did they effectively control their fertility? These questions bear little resemblance to those usually raised by sociologists of reproduction; they imply in-depth analysis, personal accounts, and the probing of motivation. Such a humanistic perspective has been conspicuously absent from this branch of the sociological industry which adheres tenaciously to the 'old simple truths of positivism' (Rex 1978: 296).

Explaining childlessness

Sociologists have tended to work from the premise that if the individual is located within the social structure then his or her reproductive behaviour is explained.

> 'The family is conceived . . . as a structural entity integrated into a larger set of structural conditions (such as the kinship system, the occupational system and the pattern of economic development) and is generally seen in terms of the requirements of these larger conditions. The decisions which occur within the family with regard to size are then assumed to be responses to such conditions.'   (Walsh 1972: 51)

Structural conditions, values, and norms are seen as directly eliciting a predetermined fertility response: a theoretical position that has resulted in a mass of statistical data from which are drawn the 'correlates and determinants' of reproductive behaviour (Hawthorn 1970). Using this perspective, Peel and Carr (1975) report that the 4 per cent of their sample of 1,448 women who desired no children 'was largely found among the older women (9 per cent of those marrying at 30 years or older), among the wives of divorced men (11 per cent), among the better-educated (10 per cent of the college-trained) and among those without religious affiliations (14 per cent). This preference existed rather more often among higher status women (7 per cent of wives of professional men and managers and similarly 7 per cent of wives of white-collar workers) than among wives of skilled manual workers (3 per cent). It was hardly found at all among the wives of other manual workers (0.4 per cent)' (p. 41). Similar findings have been reported from the United States and Canada, with the voluntarily childless disproportionately drawn from the higher status, better-educated sectors of the community (Veevers 1979).

Voluntary childlessness appears as a 'response' to a set of structural conditions. Such explanations, however, are hardly satisfying (Hawthorn 1970). Even if the connection between causal variables and rejection of parenthood is more than fortuitous, it leaves unexamined the means by which individuals with particular characteristics come to perceive their situation as necessitating a childless 'response' (Cicourel 1974). 'Normal' reproductive behaviour is assumed to be a consequence of men and women acting out the values, images, and norms they internalized during socialization and which society unambiguously attaches to parental and related institutions. Failure to conform is therefore a violation of accepted, unyielding standards: an aberration that can only be explained in terms of personal pathology or some failure in the learning process. The assumption behind such explanations of nonconformity is one of moral consensus. But to what extent does consensus characterize the reproductive framework? It has already been stressed that the empirical research which might provide an answer to this question remains to be done. But even if there is, as there appears to be, considerable agreement on the basic link between marriage and parenthood, to what extent do individuals conform blindly, willingly, quietly? Are they mere puppets, imprisoned by role-expectations, constrained by internalized norms and values? Are those who fail to conform equally constrained by their 'inadequacy' or inappropriate socialization? The view taken here is that this picture of 'oversocialized man', of a 'disembodied, conscience-driven, status-seeking phantom' (Wrong 1961: 120) is distorted. The perspective fails to 'capture the open-ended, tentative, exploratory, hypothetical, problematical, devious, changeable, and only partly unified character of courses of human action' (Strauss 1977: 91).

All individuals 'are capable of wishing to do anything and doing anything they wish' (Box 1981: 132); it is therefore simplistic and unacceptable to explain voluntary childlessness in terms of abnormality, inadequacy, or learning failure. This is not to deny that 'the world, both the natural and social world, is partially patterned, ordered and preprogrammed', but to recognize that it is also 'partially unpatterned, disordered, not preprogrammable – that experience, internal response, and action are necessarily partly contingent and free' (Douglas 1977: 61). Men and women are actors, negotiators of the social reality they inhabit and not programmed reactors at the beck and call of intransigent forces. They interpret their situation and act accordingly, therefore meanings and not structural conditions 'are in some way the fundamental determinants of social action' (Douglas 1971: 4). In other words, it is the meanings individuals attach to parenthood and related institutions within the context of their own lives that determine their reproductive activity. They have the capacity to do, think, and believe the unexpected. As Allport states:

'While we accept certain cultural values as propriate, as important for our own course of becoming, it is equally true that we are all rebels, deviants and individualists. Some elements in our culture we reject altogether; many we adopt as mere opportunistic habits, and even those elements that we genuinely appropriate we refashion to fit our own personal style of life. Culture is a condition of becoming but is not itself the full stencil.'   (Allport 1955: 82)

Individuals become what they are as their life histories unfold. It would, of course, be a gross distortion to suggest that this unfolding process is in all circumstances haphazard and unscheduled. There may not be a blue-print guiding their every step but there is often a regularity and sameness about the lives they lead. Instrumental to, and a product of, this tendency to habitualize is the cultural backcloth of values, institutions, expectations, and images that are internalized during the socialization process, subsequently taken for granted, automatically enacted, and remaining apparently immune to any expression of doubt or dissension. It is seemingly almost impossible to escape from the normal way of doing things (Brittan 1973). Shared meanings and assumptions and prescribed ways of doing and being may therefore appear fixed and immutable – an external constraint upon the social actor who is led through the routines of marriage and parenthood, following the timetabled course for legitimate parenthood: courtship-marriage-delay-conception-pregnancy-birth-delay-conception-pregnancy-birth.

Individuals have fixed ideas; they develop perspectives and routines and become committed to courses of action. But even within the confines of their limited horizons they remain actors, thinking, self-reflexive beings. Their passivity is illusory, for they actively participate in the forging of their particular social worlds (Blumer 1969; Berger and Luckmann 1967). Even in infancy children are not mere reflectors of their environment (Skolnick 1978). Although many people may choose to be and do the normal, they are not simply ciphers for convention:

'the moral sense and life-styles of most people reach far beyond the confines of domestic and community mores in which they were first fashioned. If we look into ourselves we observe that our tribal morality seems to us somehow peripheral to our personal integrity. True, we observe conventions of modesty, decorum, and self-control, and have many habits that fashion us in part as mirror-images of our home, class and cultural ways of living. But we know that we have selected, reshaped and transcended these ways to a marked degree.'   (Allport 1955: 34–5)

Nor can the 'normal' road be assumed to be without anxiety and doubt. To choose this way may be an exacting and painful task (Plummer 1975). Research has documented parenthood as 'crisis', as a threat to the mental and physical welfare of parent and child, as a stultifier of life-chances, as a task demanding undue sacrifice and begrudging obligation (Pohlman 1973). But whatever choice is made represents commitment: 'What happens is that the individual, as a consequence of actions he has taken in the past or the operation of various institutional routines, finds he must adhere to certain lines of behaviour, because many other activities than the one he is immediately engaged in will be adversely affected if he does not' (Becker 1963: 27). The man or woman who marries may repress the desire to remain childless, because to do otherwise might jeopardize not only the marital relationship but also wider family ties and reputation within the community at large. By marrying, individuals commit themselves to parenthood; they may not be attached to this position, that is, value the self-image it engenders (Goffman 1961), but having estimated the consequences of any contemplated change as too costly, will proceed to become even further entrenched.

Commitments, by limiting alternative futures, act as turning-points in the emergence of a particular career (restricted in this context to the 'changes over time as are basic and common to the members of a social category' (Goffman 1968: 119)). In relation to parenthood, marriage is an important, if not the most important turning-point in the reproductive career; it is a commitment to reproduction. Therefore, those who marry but choose to remain childless are side-stepping conventional expectations and forging alternative careers. The concern here is with the process by which a marriage becomes childless; the aim is to trace, describe and analyse, and approach an understanding of the childless career from individual inception through to the construction and management of a shared commitment. How 78 individuals, representatives of 44 couples living in and around a major Scottish city during 1974/5, became, and what it means to them to be, voluntarily childless constitutes the broad remit for this exploratory study. This is a somewhat parochial interest but, as earlier suggested, one that has implications for those 'disturbed' by the low levels of fertility in Western societies. Tracing the reproductive careers of the voluntarily childless will provide knowledge not only of the situations and meanings that inform their commitment but also of the norms, values, and images of the cultural framework. If parenthood has sustained its inevitable and desirable status, then the childless will be expected to explain their deviant behaviour but will be unable to do so except in the negative terms of pro-natalist ideology. If, on the other hand, there has been a liberalization of interpretation to allow for greater freedom of reproductive choice, then their decision will go unchallenged but be supported by a vocabulary of motives (Mills 1940) that will both inform and maintain their commitment. Voluntary childlessness, in other words, would have become a legitimate alternative to parenthood.

2

Becoming voluntarily childless:
alternative careers

How individuals come to acquire the meanings that inform their reproductive behaviour is a complex and, as yet, only partially understood process. There is, however, evidence to suggest that 'socialization for fertility is a long-term and continuously unfolding process, with influences stemming from a multiplicity of sources that shift in relative importance over the life-cycle' (Fox, Fox, and Frohardt-Lane 1982: 45). The process begins in childhood and is strongly influenced by the form and nature of family life (Gustavus and Nam 1970; Johnson and Stokes 1976). It is hardly surprising that there exists a consistency between generations on the issue of reproductive norms; who individuals are and what they do is initially dependent upon 'chance and opportunism' and not upon their own conscious efforts (Allport 1955). As children, they have little choice in the commitments that are laid down in trust for them by those who act as the mediators between them and the pre-existing social world. During early years 'the individual's first world is constructed . . . Only later can (he/she) afford the luxury of at least a modicum of doubt' (Berger and Luckmann 1967: 156).

During childhood, individuals learn not only to cope with their immediate circumstances but also internalize, in anticipation of the future, programmes relating to the playing of adult roles (Berger and Luckmann 1967). The first stage on the road to becoming a parent is therefore traversed during primary socialization as the little girl tends to her dolls 'that not only look like real babies, but act like them' (Silverman and Silverman 1971: 17), whilst her brother dons his father's bowler and takes the 8.05 to the City. Meanings relating to femininity and masculinity, marriage and parenthood, pregnancy and child-care emerge in embryo during the interaction of parents and child and form the basis for a process of becoming that continues unabated through adolescence and on into adulthood – a process so successful as to evince reactions such as those noted by Radkin in the 1960s:

> 'Harry Harlow, the psychologist, was in San Antonio, Texas, giving a lecture that my wife and I attended. The first thing he did was to put up a picture of an ugly infant. I mean a new born monkey. It's kind of cadaverous. It doesn't have much meat on its bones. It's really honest-to-God ugly. The audience began to coo. There were a lot of college women, probably virgin, single, southwestern girls. The room sounded like a seaplane taking off, "oooh!" The room was roaring with coos. Now this is phony as hell. This is social pressure.'
> (Silverman and Silverman 1971: 14)

As it was for these girls, for many more men and women, the final denouement – becoming wife/mother, husband/father – may often be a foregone conclusion long before the possibility of actualization presents itself.

But meanings relating to adult statuses are not necessarily uniform throughout society and may vary between social groups. Malinowski's now out-dated analysis illustrates this point:

> 'In the Christian Aryan societies . . . pregnancy among the lower classes is made a burden, and regarded as a nuisance; among the well-to-do people it is a source of embarrassment, discomfort and temporary ostracism from ordinary social life.'
> (quoted in Deutsch 1945: 10)

Meanings internalized during childhood will reflect those most salient amongst the parental reference group as well as the idiosyncratic interpretation of parents themselves. Parenthood may therefore be seen as inevitable and natural by the group but defined by individual members as a burdensome, or boring, or joyful, or nondescript, natural and inevitable experience. To these embellishments must be added the further possibility – given man's propensity for the unexpected – of a divergence in interpretation on the part of either parent or child. When the former is the case, the meanings conveyed are likely to be reflected in the child's perceptions. Meanings emerging out of childhood experiences may therefore provide the impetus behind a later commitment to childlessness.

Marjorie Nelson: 'My mother she said to me, "Don't you ever have children". My mother was in labour for a fortnight, with me she suffered for a fortnight. As she said for a fortnight she cursed me she called me for everything and she kept saying, "I wish I'd never had it". Whether it is transferable, I just don't know. If such a thing is possible – that something can be planted in the mind of an unborn baby then I reckon, yes, it has happened. I don't see how any child can be so adamant all the way through its life even when it's tiny. To turn round and say you don't want a brother or sister, you just want a pup . . . every child I've come across has wanted a brother or sister.'

Parental influence is not always so obvious and direct (Fox, Fox, and Frohardt-Lane 1982); simply by their actions parents may place children in situations which appear to engender the emergence of meanings that facilitate questioning of the inevitability and desirability of the 'family ideal'. Only children and those from homes in which parents appear as 'martyrs' to their role have already been identified as disproportionately represented amongst the childless (Veevers 1979; Campbell 1984); it seems likely that the growing number of adults and children living in contexts other than the nuclear unit will be instrumental in producing a more equivocal interpretation of family life and a more liberal evaluation of what up to now have been seen as undesirable alternatives. This is not, however, to suggest that there will be an automatic increase in childlessness. Children may accept and desire to adhere to what is 'normal' according to the public image even when parents openly advise otherwise (Johnson and Stokes 1976).

Important though it would appear to be, the interaction of

parent and child during primary socialization is only one amongst a number of sources from which meanings informing childless commitment may emerge. Socialization is a life-long process (Brim 1966); at the age of 19, the six-year-old who was categorical in her desire for babies may look forward with less certainty to the maternal role. A host of potential socializing agents exist either to reinforce or to subvert meanings internalized during childhood. A recently emergent source of unconventional ideas on family, marriage, and motherhood has been the modern feminist movement. Initially rejected as overly militant by many men and women, its less strident demands of the 1970s have struck a more concordant note particularly amongst adolescent women whose socialization for motherhood is still in progress (Bernard 1975b). Obviously not all young women are versed in the feminist debate, nor perceive it as relevant to their future lives, but 'by now it has probably influenced all women in the western world whether they like it or not and whether they know it or not' (Dally 1982: 165). Contemporary adolescents, admittedly highly-educated with favourable career prospects, do not wish to become 'the martyred, self-sacrificing traditional mother'. They 'rarely ask the old marriage-versus-career question now. More and more they ask instead, What else am I going to do besides being a mother? They take the else for granted' (Bernard 1975b: 91). They believe that women should not subordinate themselves to men, that men should participate equally in household tasks, that adequate child-care facilities should be provided outside the home. They are, Bernard argues, 'being socialized for a style of motherhood consonant with the times'.

'Times' change and the young woman facing adulthood may find herself at odds with parents, particularly her mother, who, at her age, faced a different future:

'My mother feels I should go to college and the first week I'm out of college I should marry some guy and have six kids . . . I'd like to work for a while first. Maybe I'd . . . get good at it, get a decent salary. Then maybe I'd think about getting married. Just so I'd accomplish something. Not just to be a woman so you can have babies and perpetuate life.'

(Bernard 1975b: 92)

This hypothetical life-plan reflects to a certain extent the superficiality of much feminist thinking on the question of motherhood. Feminists have tended to trivialize the maternal role and to downgrade its joys, benefits, and responsibilities whilst failing to 'identify true maternal devotion and to encourage it, or to study the varieties of motherhood that are needed in the modern world or the kinds that are likely to be needed in the future' (Dally 1982: 184). They aim to 'liberate' women, in this case from the 'Myth of Motherhood', to allow them freely to choose a reproductive option: a goal hardly enhanced by the cavalier and often hostile way in which the 'problem' of mothers and children is approached. In *The Female Eunuch* (1971), Germaine Greer was highly critical of conventional motherhood yet unwilling to renounce the possibility of having children; 'I thought of the children I knew in Calabria and hit upon the plan to buy, with the help of some friends with similar problems, a farmhouse in Italy where we could stay when circumstances permitted, and where our children would be born. Their fathers and other people would also visit the house as often as they could, to rest and enjoy the children . . . Being able to be with my child and his friends would be a privilege and delight that I could work for' (p. 235). Firestone (1972), however, sees nothing positive in the experience; pregnancy is like 'shitting a pumpkin . . . the temporary deformation of the body of the individual for the sake of the species' (pp. 188–89). She demands that women be freed from the tyranny of reproduction and that child-care be the responsibility of society as a whole. These antipathetic and, at times, hysterical statements are unlikely to gain credence amongst the mass of women and have indeed been somewhat tempered; what has filtered through, however, is a diluted version that rejects the idea of motherhood as the *sine qua non* of a woman's existence and goes so far as to suggest that women who perform none other than the wife/mother role are potential victims of mental/emotional deprivation: in popular parlance they become 'cabbages', household drudges, 'just housewives'. There appears to be little sympathy or tolerance for the woman who becomes steeped in the 'trivia' of child-care. According to one childless woman who shared this perspective, her female friends had 'been fairly alive, intelligent people and then all of a sudden they get pregnant, they have a kid and they just turn into these sort of nappy-talking bores. It's really frightening because these are people I've talked to for hours and they've been interesting people. They can see it themselves, it's upsetting for them as well as for me, but they just don't seem to be able to talk about anything else except the brat.'

This unofficial interpretation of motherhood as 'possession' and 'self-sacrifice' offers a counterbalance to the public image and provides justification for the childless decision.

Whatever the source of disaffection from the reproductive norm, an adolescent, cognisant of parenthood's darker side, to become voluntarily childless must translate this knowledge into the desire to avoid parenthood and the desire into the opportunity (Box 1981). Of the 78 respondents, 17 women and 13 men had followed this career, becoming childless before meeting their prospective marriage partners. Any commitment to avoidance depends upon individuals seeing such a course of action as in their interest; this is unlikely to be a rational calculation at this stage and may reach consciousness as a straightforward, unarticulated rejection of parenthood. One of the respondents, Tom Irvine, said: 'I could make a case and it would all look jolly nice as a Sunday *Observer Review* . . . but it would not in fact be true. I just don't know (why); I've always felt that way.' Not everyone who wants to avoid parenthood, will do so; during childhood and adolescence commitment to childlessness has little relevance for daily existence and deviant intentions go unnoticed or, if articulated, are perceived as adolescent rebellion. Relevance becomes apparent when the question of marriage arises. Marriage implies parenthood and may therefore be seen as incompatible with childless commitment (Veevers 1980).

Sheila Kidd: 'I'm 27 and I've only been married two months. We'd known each other about six-and-a-half years. I just didn't want to get married before because I had this thing about my job and, as I say, I was quite definite that I didn't want children.'

Those who reject the feasibility of marriage are acting upon the assumption that parenthood is the 'natural' *sequitur* and that they themselves are in some sense 'odd' or 'abnormal'; the possibility of marriage appears remote (Veevers 1980). A prospective partner might even be the catalyst that brings to consciousness an individual's wish to remain childless. Three respondents, including Sandra O'Neill, had experienced this transformation (Berger and Luckmann 1967).

Sandra O'Neill: 'I used to go around with this bloke before I met Jimmy and he was an only child and his big ambition was to get married and have a big family. And he said this to me and it immediately turned me right off, just something said, "No, you don't want a lot of children, if you want any at all".'

Where conventional interpretations of marriage and parenthood have been rejected and individuals see themselves as acting quite legitimately, marriage is simply a question of finding like-minded partners: a search they see as no more arduous than that pursued by the reproductively 'normal'.

Hilary Dexter: 'I had certainly (considered childlessness before marriage) . . . it hadn't occurred to me that I could ever meet anyone I would want to marry who wouldn't share my views . . . It's principally how I've felt since I was 20.'

Alan Dexter: 'I think my views formed much earlier . . . I just know it would be a disaster if I ever had children . . . When I was 16 I began thinking like this . . . We'd discussed it (prior to marriage), before we'd even slept together and agreed straightaway.'

Commitment to childlessness is shared, therefore; although meanings informing the decision may vary, the definition of any future marriage is fixed. Some reinterpretation does take place, bringing divergent cases more into line, but given the shared centrality of remaining childless for both partners and the extent of self-validation this entails, once they have formed a common front, variations in interpretation may be accepted and supported even if not always espoused. Thirteen women and 12 men had been able to find like-minded partners.

Where reproductive intentions vary, the relationship may end or continue with the childless capitulating to normality or attempting to persuade the other to accept marriage without children; four women and one man had successfully taken the latter course. The outcome will depend primarily upon strength of original commitment and the perceived costs and benefits of conversion; conversion may be immediate or a lengthy process taking a number of years and the marriage be postponed until both partners are convinced of the other's intentions.

Liz Finlay: 'When we got married Alan knew that I never had any intention, I just didn't want children.'

Interviewer: 'So you'd told him, had you, before?'

Liz Finlay: 'Oh yes.'

Interviewer: 'What had his reaction been?'

Liz Finlay: 'If you don't want them, you don't want them. And I'd said "Would you come along (to interview)?" and he said "What's the point, if you want children to-morrow, we'll have children to-morrow".'

Sheila Kydd: 'Sometimes I think, well, maybe it's a bit selfish to have this attitude but, well, he knew that when we married so it's not as if . . .'

Donald Kydd: 'Sprung it on me, no.'

Interviewer: 'What was your reaction when you first knew?'

Donald Kydd: 'When I first heard it I said she's joking. I actually said that. I said, "You must be joking". That was my exact words . . . after that I realized she was serious. I must admit I had to have a long think about it . . . I love kids. And I had a long think about it and I think . . . well, every man likes to have a son, I suppose, as the saying goes. But after a couple of years, three years, two and a half years, I felt that she was really serious. Before I used to say, "Aye, aye, I'll accept it, I know you don't want kids".'

Sheila Kydd: 'Even till . . . when we got engaged I said no children. I don't think you really believed me when I told you then. You kept on thinking, "Oh, she'll change her mind".'

Donald Kydd: 'I didn't say that. It started off as she'll change her mind, then she might change her mind. Maybe she'll not, then she won't. That was the stage it went through.'

Having to assume a socializing role may leave one partner feeling he/she has pressurized the other into accepting a role for which he/she has no genuine desire and that acceptance will be subsequently revoked. These fears may persist even where the previously uncommitted become attached to their childless identity and wholeheartedly espouse the childless way of life. So complete a conversion is rarely evident. Agreement may be reached but be accompanied by no more than a conditional commitment. Commitment is specific to the present relationship; if this was to break down, parenthood for the converted might become a viable alternative. Donald Kydd: 'nobody knows what the future holds. If something happened to Sheila and I was left alone, you never know I might get married again. I might want kids . . .' The working definition of the marriage as childless may simply paper over the rarely articulated, yet deep divisions that persist between husband and wife on questions relating to parenthood; but what is certain is that the couple, while they remain together, are to be childless; this is the all-important concession upon which the relationship stands or falls and from which the joint career takes its starting-point.

Not all childless careers begin before marriage; of the respondents, 26 men and 19 women had become childless after marriage. Childlessness may be a product of, as well as a prerequisite for, marital interaction. Post-marital commitment tends to be extended, at times spasmodic (Veevers 1980): a series of actions, some fragmented and oblique, that gradually jell into acceptance of life without children.

Cathy McCormack: 'It just developed'.
Bob McCormack: 'It just developed like most of the things that happen to us . . . We didn't consciously say, "Let's have a heart-breaking talk whether to have children".'

The decision will often entail the curtailment of a prior commitment to parenthood. Taken for granted, the latter lurks in the back of the mind, rarely reaching consciousness. Before marriage couples gave little thought to family intentions; 18 of the 26 did, however, discuss parenthood in a vague and cursory way, sentiments expressed adhering more or less to conventional lines, lacking enthusiasm as well as detail, and being eclipsed by the more pressing demands of becoming a married couple.

Mike Vernon: 'We were discussing whether we should buy or rent (property) I mean that was much more the topic of conversation before we got married than children.'

Parenthood is not an immediate concern; as a status to be achieved 'some time in the future', it barely stirs the imagination. When questioned before marriage most people will express the view that they expect and hope to become parents (Dunnel 1979). There is, however, some doubt as to the sincerity and depth of anticipatory feelings toward the parental role (LeMasters 1970). Amongst the childless the tendency to mimic conventional expectations and imagery supports this view.

Carol Blair: 'Yes, (we discussed children), not in the sort of definite "We'll have children in so many years", or anything like that. We just sort of vaguely mentioned we wanted children, I think.'
Henry Blair: 'We just took it for granted, I think, we would have children.'
Carol Blair: 'Children were always some time in the future.'

The future, however, is not open. There is a time for childbearing: a stage in the family life-cycle prescribed by the prevailing reproductive time-table. Couples who had ratified commitment to parenthood were universal in their desire to postpone the event for 'a year or two': the first stage on what Veevers has characterized as the 'postponement route to childlessness' (Veevers 1980).

Mary Fraser: 'It was a conscious decision that we wouldn't have any children, I think as most couples do, to begin with. I think like everybody else, we said, "For two years . . .", this magical figure: two years.'

The phrase, 'as most young couples do', illustrates the normality of postponement and the commonsense basis of its rationale.

Charles Quin: 'I think we both felt when we got married that it was a mistake to rush into this kind of thing too quickly . . . we felt we needed a couple of years to settle down, to do things together we might not otherwise get the opportunity to do . . . we discussed it originally as far as I remember before we got married . . . and our original intention was to wait 18 months to a couple of years.'

The statutory breathing space features prominently in the reproductive folk-wisdom of these predominantly middle-class men and women. It acts as a safety-net, a guard against irresponsible parenthood, stressing as it does the obligations individuals have not only to themselves but also to partners and unborn children. Even where the wife has already passed the age appropriate for first births, couples accept the advisability of delaying for the requisite period. On the other hand, early marriage appears to justify a postponement longer than the norm: a delay that would in fact bring the teenage bride more into line with the image of the young mother as a woman in her mid-20s. One girl, married at 18, had seen the future as follows:

Betty Hamilton: 'Like most other girls I wanted to have a family. He did at the time as well. I wanted six boys and he wanted six girls; that was only fun. There had been no decision made at the time apart from the fact that we didn't want to have children till we had both got through our courses and then worked for quite a few years.'

Although vague, imprecise, disintèrested, these decisions made and timetables drawn up prior to marriage demonstrate a recognized and shared commitment to parenthood. Eight couples however had made no attempt to interlink reproductive careers. The women involved had either expected to have children and had read a conventional interpretation into the mutual silence:

Patricia Campbell: 'No, never discussed it . . . I thought I would probably at the time as Ken was good with other people's children, and it was only when we got married that I realized it was other people's children. He did not want his own.'

or could not remember having given the question any thought.

Maggie Smith: 'I hadn't thought about it before I got married at all, not consciously. I hadn't had any desire to have children and I hadn't thought about not having any; I just hadn't thought about it at all.'

The husbands of these women had either abrogated reproductive responsibility or already committed themselves to a childless way of life; either way they saw it as an issue for the women to raise. One other couple, although considering the question independently, had come to the same conclusion: that parenthood was to be accorded no special status within the context of their relationship.

Mike Vernon: 'We never said, "Are we going to have children? Are we going to have six children? Are we going to have two children?".'

Ellen Vernon: 'I think it's never been important to either of us in a sense.'

Mike Vernon: 'We didn't get married for children, that's for sure.'

Ellen Vernon: 'We've talked to other people who've said "What's the point in getting married if you're not going to have children?" Well, thinking about that, then the answer is, yes, I did think about it before I was married and it never seemed to me to be terribly important. What was important was the relationship that two people have and whether or not one had children depended on circumstances, what you felt like, how well your job was going, but it was certainly never, you know, we never sat there holding hands, saying, "We'll have six children, three boys and three girls and won't it be lovely".'

Most couples did not recognize this degree of choice; according to the popular image, once the period of adjustment is over parenthood falls naturally into place and a harmonious family is created. Nonetheless, they did not perceive children as the apex of their life-plans. This observation supports Cicourel's contention that 'we cannot take it for granted that the focal point of family life revolves around not being able to conceive, a desire for male offspring, having "too many children", stillbirth and the like though these issues certainly intrude on some part of a family's existence' (Cicourel 1967: 59).

Couples marry expecting to become parents; they legitimately postpone pregnancy through the use of effective contraception but fail to go on and realize their reproductive intentions. Intentions are not fixed; the meanings that inform reproductive commitment may be suspended, modified, subsequently reinstated, or subverted in the course of an unfolding life history. Negative may become positive and positive become negative in the light of changing situations and interests.

Jeannie Maxwell: 'When I was first married, everyone I knew got married and had a little house and had children and I thought this was – this was all I'd been brought up to expect. Since '67 I've realized there's a much larger field. I'll be honest, if I had a child now, I'd spend the first year with it and then go back to work again. It wouldn't be sufficient for me to be at home. I would then have to have another outlet . . . I now realize my home and a child ultimately would not be enough for me.'

Charles Quin: 'I think I'd always visualized myself as a family man, pushing the pram along the street . . . I don't know, maybe it's getting older but I'm beginning to feel that being a parent isn't perhaps all that rosy. Also I've had all this worry and it's been considerable, worry over my health . . . it's been going on now for two years in July . . . I don't want Evelyn to be left with a young child to be brought up . . . I think that was the first thing that influenced me towards feeling it was a thing that should be deferred. Since then, seeing other people, thinking more about it, seeing the general state of the world.'

'Indefinite postponement' (Veevers 1980), through illness, financial worry, the desire to create a better environment in which to parent, will tend to place couples out of step with their contemporaries who have adhered more closely to the reproductive timetable. Those who remain childless are able to observe, evaluate, and compare the two life-styles; comparisons may reflect parenthood's darker side and provide the meanings that motivate childless commitment. Leslie Graham: 'I think also looking at a lot of marriages of friends of ours that have had children helped to make the decision as well . . . Not really disasters, just living together, you know, but it's a very ropy sort of thing'. 'Indefinite postponement' also allows individuals and couples to develop commitments which may eventually be interpreted as conflicting with the demands and responsibilities of parenthood. Whatever the source of conversion, accounts suggest mutuality. Neither partner accepts or is attributed with responsibility for the decision; 'instigators' however can be identified. 'Instigators', either through word or deed, demonstrate their ambiguity towards the parental role and set the process of becoming childless into motion. Tentative overtures may be met with immediate enthusiasm, particularly where negative interpretations of parenthood have been suppressed.

Kate Tennant: 'I've always disliked babies . . . when we got married, I thought in two years I'll have a baby 'cos that's what happens when you get married . . . Then as time went by we decided – it just sort of happened – we didn't. I'm very glad we haven't a child . . . I've always, always as long as I can remember hated babies'.

From these and more cautious beginnings, the process of becoming childless may occur almost imperceptibly: a gradual process running smoothly with limited discussion, little conscious thought, rare glimpses of heart-searching and seldom an identifiable catalyst. Claire MacDonald: 'We didn't sit down . . . and discuss it. It wasn't sort of, "What do you think? What about parents, you know, what kind of education can we give our child?" I mean we haven't sort of sat down and discussed it like that'. Seldom is the issue broached head-on prior to a couple's recognition of the reciprocal nature of their commitment; any balance-sheet of the pros and cons of childlessness they draw up seems to act as *post hoc* justification and not, as Veevers has suggested (1980), as a necessary stage in the emergence of the joint career.

But not all those who become childless after marriage 'drift' into the situation: during or after the postponement period, couples who now recognize their eligibility may deliberately set out to decide whether or not to have children. They reject notions of inevitability and universal desirability; the question is, 'Do *we* want children?', a question not easily answered.

Helen Donaldson: 'The trouble is, it's much more difficult nowadays in that you do make decisions whereas before it was . . . I would certainly not want to go back to the stage where you reproduce a child a year, like my grandmother did, but certainly it does make it more of a . . . you can turn it into what I suppose we've turned it into which is an insoluble problem, if you think about it long enough.'

Deciding to remain childless depends upon a shared neutrality towards parenthood; individuals are quick to report that if their partners had 'desperately wanted children', then they 'would have had children'. In the vacuum in which they find themselves, husband and wife act as mutual socializing agents; pointing out the pros and cons of alternative careers and asking, 'What do *we* want to do with *our* lives?' They do not accept the inevitability and universal desirability of parenthood's public image and feel under no moral pressure to conform. These are men and women who share the feminist demand for freedom of reproductive choice.

Husband and wife do not always develop parallel reproductive careers. Values and intentions may be diametrically opposed: one partner may wish to remain childless, the other to have children; the situation is an obvious source of conflict.

Joan Ellison: 'I brought it up about the fact that some day we might have a family but my husband was the first to suggest that why should we or need we – he questions everything and I think when he put his point of view I quite agree really and I'm really pleased now to think we didn't rush into this sort of decision.'
Interviewer: 'What was your first reaction?'
Joan Ellison: 'Possibly horror because I would be a bit worried about what people would think in the first place.'

This study included only three cases of conflicting commitment and therefore no conclusions can be drawn as to how couples

resolve such dilemmas, but the facility with which the conventionally committed accept the childless alternative highlights the
ongoing nature of reproductive socialization and the ease with
which likely pressure can be minimized when couples share
deviant intentions. Once a couple have committed themselves to
childlessness, the joint career is under way. Together they begin
to create a way of life that becomes increasingly dependent upon
the maintenance of their childless commitment. Attachment,
where previously absent, may develop to reinforce a commitment that gradually becomes taken for granted.

Maggie Smith: 'In the early years one was conscious of not
wanting children then – after a time it became a habit, to avoid
both the begetting of children and children themselves. We do
not encourage children around us – we never invite people to
bring their children to the house. And with us in general,
children have not been considered as part of life – my husband
has gazed wistfully on fabulous cars in magazines, on the
roads, on films – and I have done the same with houses,
clothes, holidays – it is almost in some ways as though children
don't exist – they are something which other people have . . .
But it has never occurred to us to emulate them. If it were not
for the chance that one could "contract" children oneself like a
disease which is almost how we regard it – you, as it were,
wash your hands thoroughly because you do not want to get
something to make you ill, but you do not spend hours
discussing the possibility of measles or infection – and for the
fact that they are around everywhere and other couples have
them, I don't think they would have been thought of at all . . . I
think that even in the early years, had it not been for the fact
that one was well aware that normal relationships seemed to
go – engagement, marriage, home, children – the topic might
never have been mentioned at all with mutual silent agreement that neither of us wanted them.'

Commitment to a course of action however is never foreclosed
until irreversible. A woman's commitment to childlessness, for
example, may be revoked to the point where she is either
sterilized or finds herself overtaken by the menopause when
what was previously a question of choice becomes one of

inevitability – even then the possibility of surrogate motherhood remains. Individuals vary and couples do not always agree on the extent of their commitment (Veevers 1980); they may be certain that childlessness is the most desirable option now and for the foreseeable future but be unwilling to commit themselves indefinitely.

Betty Oliver: 'I'm keeping options open, I think I've got to . . . I know I've changed a lot from when I was 16 to now, so I could change a lot from now till I'm 30 . . . I still have my doubts, not because I'm pressurized but because I'm terrified that I'll change my mind.'

Just over half the respondents, equally divided between men and women, shared this 'provisional' commitment; the remainder saw their commitment as 'total': they could envisage no circumstance in which they might change their minds.

Betty Hamilton: 'I can't see any reason to make me change my mind in the future . . . I think as I get older my attitude will become more and more definite, People don't seem to realize that once you have made up your mind to do something, then that's it, I feel I am making the right decision.'

Degree of commitment influences the way individuals and couples cope with one of the recurring problems of the childless career: preventing accidental pregnancy. 'Total' commitment allows consideration of a once-and-for-all solution: sterilization. The desire to foreclose options – to become voluntarily sterile – has been linked to timing of commitment; 'early articulators' (Houseknecht 1978), those making premarital commitment, individuals who 'felt that "being a parent is not for me",' were found to favour sterilization (Veevers 1980: 29). This study does not support this finding. Timing of the decision does appear to be related to its basis: pre-marital commitment tends to result from rejection of parenthood, post-marital from acceptance of childlessness, but rejection of parenthood does not predispose towards 'total' commitment and sterilization. 'Rejectors' never having seen themselves as parents are, however, more likely to accept abortion as a solution to unwanted pregnancy.

Unwanted pregnancy is not the only threat to childless commitment; couples must also face the problem of living within a cultural climate that, if it does not condemn, does not condone voluntary childlessness. They may take their situation for granted but rarely do outsiders allow them to forget the fact that they have no children. If they had become parents, they would not have been expected to explain or justify their conformity to reproductive normality (Mills 1940); parenthood is the 'natural' *sequitur* to marriage and therefore goes unchallenged. Remaining childless beyond the postponement period is out of the ordinary – if not abnormal – and liable to demands for explanation. Reproduction is still a 'public' issue; privatization of family life appears not to have eliminated the right of the wider community to demand an explanation for those who deviate from the public image (Stycos 1958). But even before explanations are requested, couples may be subject to pressure, both direct and indirect, from peers who have already become parents (Waller and Hill 1951). As friends and acquaintances around them 'leave' to become mothers, women in particular may believe that this is what they should do in spite of doubts to the contrary.

Barbara Hargraves: 'A colleague who works along at the end was saying that his wife was a teacher and she wasn't sure whether she particularly wanted children but she kept seeing colleagues leaving term after term and having children. It was the accepted thing.'

Women who marry with a childless clause in the 'contract' (Veevers 1980), although not immune to pressure, recognize the source of their uncertainty and are able to reaffirm their commitment with their husbands' support.

Ellen Kennedy: 'Well, Roy had decided he didn't want children and I had really decided . . . I didn't give children a thought before I was married and I don't know whether it is because of society but I sometimes think now, would I like a family, am I missing out on a family? But, I mean really, before we got married we decided, we'd both decided individually, of course, because we didn't know one another, I mean, I always said if I got married, I didn't want a family and Roy's the same . . . Mind you, you get it drummed into you continually that this is what marriage is all about. When I'd been married three months my boss came up to me and said, "Have you got your resignation in yet?" I said, "No". He said, "I'd have thought you'd have had it in by now". I said, "Given my own way, I'll not have any at all". He was taken aback, I think. Society does tend to think are you not having a family. It's amazing the people that . . . either that or they'll sort of indiscreetly say, "What age are you?". You say, "Twenty-five", and they think to themselves, "She'd better hurry up and get a move on". Again most of the women I work with, they've come back from having their families, and they tend to think, you know, you can see it when they say something to you, they don't condemn you but at times they're a bit cruel . . . just with their inference . . . they make you out that you're just working for the money which I suppose you really are working for but you're not forsaking a baby just for the fact that you're wanting the money. I mean you're forsaking a baby because you don't want that sort of life . . . I honestly wouldn't like to say, I wouldn't say just now I'm going to be childless for all my life. I suppose you've got to swither. I mean I feel it's born in them, I think a motherly instinct . . . I don't know whether I'm being forced to feel that way; if people left me in peace I probably wouldn't think of it, or get doubts . . . when you get doubts, you tend to say, "Do you really want a child," or is it because people are . . .'

Roy Kennedy: 'How often have you said when we've left your mother's, when your sister's been there with the kids and we've been driving home and you'll say, "Definitely, that's it, no kids" . . . No, I won't change my mind.'

Ellen Kennedy: 'If he never changes his mind, I won't, 'cos as I say I wouldn't have a child without the two of us wanting it . . .'

Couples whose post-marital commitment follows protracted postponement do not register pressure as relevant to their situation. They would have conformed, but 'fate' intervened and now they are 'too old'. Age does not forestall criticism, but there is a suitable age for parenthood (Rindfuss and Bumpass 1976) and having missed this, women in particular use their advancing years to excuse their persistent non-conformity.

Excuses are not available for those whose decision is a rational acceptance of the childless alternative made during or just after the postponement period. They develop a repertoire of parrying tactics (See Chapter 6) but may also find themselves in sympathetic surroundings.

Barbara Hargraves: 'There are a lot of women here who work, who don't have children, who are perfectly happy . . .'

James Hargraves: 'Your assistant, Liz, said she'd much rather have her cat.'

Barbara Hargraves: 'But I think where the pressure isn't definitely upon you and where it isn't considered the norm to trot round having children then you consider yourself very much more carefully what it is that you want, and what you should be doing in the circumstances. It's certainly not the norm here to leave . . . to go round having children. You're not expected to do it, therefore you feel free to do your own thing. I think it takes a lot of pressure off you where it isn't considered the norm. They do "glug" slightly over babies when they're brought in but it isn't the same adoration and feeling of "How marvellous".'

Individuals working in higher education and research organizations report the least critical reactions. Where situations are not so favourable, couples may attempt to create a more supportive environment by 'dropping' censorious friends and cultivating the acquaintance of individuals who appear to accept the validity of their assumptions, even if they do not live by them.

The longer a couple remains childless, the more secure their commitment. After 10 years of marriage, they appear immune to adverse comment; this is not to say their decision is now immutable. Many women, whose decision was 'provisional', expressed some anxiety as to how they would feel during their mid-to-late-thirties as the menopause approached. Unfortunately only a few women had faced this situation and had made either a 'total' commitment some years ago or believed themselves incapable of conceiving. It is possible that when women do reach this 'critical' period, they will find support for their childlessness from the reproductive timetable: older mothers are more likely to give birth to defective infants and they may, as the folk wisdom suggests, find it more difficult to cope with the heavy physical and emotional demands of bearing and rearing children. But neither timetable nor folk-wisdom are static; if the trend towards later first births continues (OECD 1979), the period of eligibility may be expected to extend at least into the early 30s and the wider availability of screening tests for deformity, such as amniocentesis, may render late pregnancy a more acceptable alternative. The 'critical' period may become even more critical for childless women of the future.

Once the female has passed the menopause, the opportunity for natural parenthood is lost. Childlessness is now inevitable. There remains, however, one escape route: surrogate parent-hood. No couple had seriously considered this option; it did however carry symbolic importance, not, as in the case of Veevers's respondents (1980), as a means of delaying the final decision, but to forestall the doubts of individuals who felt they might experience a vacuum in their lives once they had achieved all they set out to achieve through the medium of their child-lessness and to keep open the possibility of family life to those who reject parenthood and looking after children but who would enjoy the company of a young adult.

Being without children is a fluid condition. Individuals and situations can change and with them interpretations of childless-ness. The childless career continues into middle and old age, and couples may be uncertain as to how they will perceive their decision during the latter stages of the life-cycle. Supportive role-models as described by one couple are rarely available:

James Hargraves: 'I think as long as we can continue to talk to each other and discuss everything at a partnership level we shall not run into too many problems.'

Barbara Hargraves: 'We have one pair of super friends, he's 77 and she must be heading for the 70s. He's a retired consultant surgeon ... she went to London University and has done social work and has done various different things in literary work. She's the daughter of a professor. And they're as happy as sand boys together. They've obviously got what's another good working partnership. They have their minor discussions but they're completely self-contained. They've got through to a ripe old age of well past 70, still doing everything together and still obviously so complete without any gaps in their life . . . And they don't have any family. And that's an example of a couple who do run well together.'

Others either prepare themselves for or reject the possibility of loneliness, a spectre readily conjured up by their critics.

Susan Dobie: 'At the back of my mind there is John's health. I don't expect him to live on to a late age so I prepare myself for that. I think I'll be on my own for quite a while afterwards. I daresay I'll be left on my own as I won't have any relations by that age either. If I do have a family they'll move away and get married. So you're back to square one. It's selfish to have a family as insurance for old age. I'm such an independent person anyway that by the time that comes along I'll adapt quite easily.'

3

Avoiding parenthood:
formative experiences of youth

The wish to avoid parenthood can be traced back to childhood and adolescence (Houseknecht 1978); why it emerged is less easily identified (Veevers 1980). The adult, asked to justify a youthful commitment, may recall only a general antipathy towards the parental role: 'I just didn't want to live like that'; 'I just knew it wasn't for me'. This lack of specificity is not solely attributable to loss of memory or to unwillingness to 'tell the truth'. Individuals who become parents may be equally vague about their motivation (Busfield and Paddon 1977). The parent and the youthful 'non-conformist' share one thing in common: neither are required to justify their reproductive intentions. Legitimate parenthood and single childlessness go un-challenged. Only when individuals find themselves in situ-ations that question the validity of, or require them to act upon, their intentions, may they come to articulate their motives (Mills 1940). For those wishing to avoid parenthood, the con-templation of marriage, the making of career decisions, choice of a form of contraception, financial commitments, the observation of peers becoming parents, may all create conditions that lead to the construction of a case against parenthood. By this time, however, the meanings that emerged out of the observations, encounters, and relationships of childhood and adolescence and that informed the initial stages of the childless career may have become obsolete, redundant, and beyond immediate recall. Adult experiences and the meanings they provoke provide a source of new motives that may supplant the original, frequently barely articulated motives that no longer have relevance for the adult. But although the roots of youthful commitment may lie buried in an irretrievable past, meanings that informed its early, if not initial stages, can be gleaned from anecdotes and stories conjured up out of childhood memories.

Marjorie Nelson: 'Even my cousins used to get me annoyed. I always felt – I was five before my first cousin arrived – to me they were stupid and babyish. They were just ridiculous – the things they used to want to do – I had grown past that stage, I'd never really done that sort of thing anyhow, to me, to sit in the middle of a mud puddle and get covered in mud was just not on. I suppose in a way I just wasn't a child.'

Meanings that do remain central to individual commitment as motives of considerable weight appear to be the product of encounters and experiences so vivid in the actor's pictorial biography as to be ineradicable.

Jim McCausland: 'the worst thing working-class people can do is have families . . . I was brought up in a very depressed working-class family . . . I think that's basically why I never wanted to have children . . . you're no giving yourself a chance and you're no giving your kid a chance . . . you're cutting your throat, you're beating your head to a pulp.'

Veevers (1980) warns against accepting such statements at face value:

'It is important to emphasize at this point that our interviews relied heavily on retrospective perceptions which, of course, are significantly affected by one's current life situation. Thus, it is quite likely that our respondents' impressions of their formative years were guided, at least in part, by what has happened subsequent to those years. It is possible that some respondents may have overemphasized their "troubled" family life in order to justify their present childfree life-style, which radically differs from that of their own parents. *Post hoc* justifications of family size are difficult to interpret in terms of cause and effect.'   (p. 39–40)

All views of the past are of necessity selective: therefore it is hardly surprising that individuals attempting to make sense of and articulate their early experience should highlight influences outside their immediate control. This tendency to 'escape blame' may be particularly marked amongst the voluntarily childless since there exists no socially approved motive for their action: 'At the present time, for a woman to come out openly against motherhood in principle is physically dangerous. She can get away with it only if she adds that she is neurotic, abnormal, child-hating and therefore "unfit" ' (Firestone 1972: 190). Motives may be tailored to fit situations. Social scientists have tended to stress the role of conditions external to the individual when explaining deviant behaviour. In the interview, 'inadequate family background' may be proffered as the motive most likely to gain acceptance; respondents in this study tended not to overplay this card even when apparently justified. The presence of a spouse, who might be expected to have detailed knowledge of a partner's past, may have checked the use of such *post hoc* justifications. This may also have been the reason why individuals were quick to point out that situations they believed favoured their decision – childhood poverty, the world situation, overpopulation – had not motivated *their* action but were nevertheless 'relevant facts' for the case against parenthood. A similar distinction was drawn between motives that had informed initial commitment and those that had subsequently emerged. The latter were not considered in the same light as 'relevant facts', since they were perceived as instrumental in the maintenance of commitment.

Motives emerge out of situations. No one situation will invariably produce meanings to motivate avoidance of parenthood. To understand childlessness, however, it is necessary to identify situations that provide individuals with the opportunity to consider careers other than the parental. In other words, which situations favour negative interpretation of parenthood? This information can only be gleaned from detailed observation of individual biographies (Blumer 1969; Douglas 1971).

The exercise is, of necessity, intuitive: 'in some way we must rely upon our understanding of everyday life, gained through direct observations of that life and *always* involving the use of our own commonsense understandings derived from our direct involvements in it' (Douglas 1971: 4). The researcher, however, must be always open to modify her commonsense under-standings in the light of observations of the 'alien' social world. This is a far from simple remit: 'It is a tough job requiring a high order of careful and honest probing, creative yet disciplined imagination, resourcefulness and flexibility in study, pondering over what one is finding and a constant readiness to test and retest one's views and images of the area' (Blumer 1969: 40). The result is an attempt to link biographical episodes to meanings that inform the desire to avoid parenthood and to the transformation of this desire into childless marriage.

Parenthood as loss of control over self and future

Sacrifice is a feature of the parental, but more specifically of the maternal role: mothers are expected to provide 'constant attention night and day, seven days a week and 365 days in the year . . . In no other relationship do human beings place them-selves so unreservedly and so continuously at the disposal of others' (Bowlby 1967: 77–78). This loss of control over self and future was the most frequently cited motive for wishing to avoid parenthood. Parents were described as 'losing control'; children as taking over and pulling the strings, jolting the parent into immediate, gratificatory action.

Elaine Morrison: 'We (colleagues) discuss it . . . I say, "How are you going to get up every single night? How are you going to get on for the first five years? Your life is manoeuvred by somebody else". And they say, "But you don't feel it, it will pass". But things don't just pass . . . I don't want to sacrifice that way.'

Many women may accept selfless action as a 'natural' price to pay for the satisfaction and enjoyment children bring, but there will also be others who resent and are cowed by the constant demands of child-care (Oakley 1982). The majority of re-spondents, born during the 1940s and 50s when the belief in the primacy of the mother-child bond was at its strongest, describe the role of full-time home-maker and child-minder, as played by their mothers, as having been in their own but not their mothers' interests. Comparisons drawn between mothers as they are now – 'childfree' – and as they were when carrying the responsibilities of motherhood, are used to emphasize the point.

Jane Archer: 'I'm the eldest of four, the youngest in the family was born when I was 11 . . . my younger brother is still only 15, and my mother having just got rid of us, realized what wonderful things one can do when you don't have children around . . . I think it got a bit much a lot of times . . . once we started to grow up she got young again. She realized there were other things in life.'

Mothers were 'always there', a fact the desirability of which mothers themselves may later come to question.

Carol Thompson: 'My mother always said if she had a life to live again she wouldn't be married and have children . . . she said she would like freedom; not to be tied down . . . it wasn't until very recently – the last year that my mother's actually come out and said this.'

The era of the 'child as king' may have passed its zenith (Ariès 1980); but nevertheless considerable obstacles, both practical and emotional, face the woman who seeks personal fulfilment through a combination of roles that includes, but does not elevate, the maternal. Oakley (1982) cites at some length the tragic case of the poet, Sylvia Plath, as an extreme example of the way in which women as wives and mothers can lose control over themselves, their talents, and their futures.

'It is so frustrating to feel that with time to study and work lovingly at my books I could do something considerable, while now I have my back to the wall and not even time to read a book . . . I just haven't felt to have any identity under the steamroller of decisions and responsibilities of this last year, with the babies a constant demand . . .

How I would like to be self-supporting on my writing. But I need time.'   (Sylvia Plath, quoted in Oakley 1982: 68)

Loss of control, once recognized as a feature of the parental role, becomes a significant argument for its rejection. A third of all childless women saw motherhood as a threat to their identity: mothers were described as 'cabbages' buried beneath the trivia of childbearing and childrearing. Although acting as justi- fication for a decision taken on alternative grounds, this descrip- tion of the selfless, almost invisible woman is nevertheless a powerful image reinforcing commitment to childlessness.

The women most likely to accept this image of 'oppression' and 'sacrifice' tended to believe that a mother's primary responsibility is to provide continuous care 'seven days a week and 365 in the year' and that such commitment excludes the simultaneous pursuit of other goals and ambitions (Veevers 1980). Not all childless women endorse the exclusivity of motherhood. One woman quoted earlier who recognized and sympathized with the stultifying effects motherhood had had upon her mother, believed she could avoid a similar fate by continuing to pursue her career whilst adequately performing the maternal role. She admitted there might be problems, mainly organizational, but believed these could be surmounted, particularly since she had already witnessed a friend's successful attempt to combine the two roles.

Jane Archer: 'What I do notice more than anything else about friends who've had children, on the whole it's women who've had jobs and given them up who've bitterly regretted it. One has this terrible sense that they are tied down . . . It's not so much being tied down that frightens me as this business . . . a child takes an awful lot of looking after. There's so much playing and talking and all the things one does with children, that there's little time for anything else. Some of them do say if only we could escape for a few hours a day just so there wasn't this constant little toddler at your side, being constantly looked after. There's just no time to think of anything else when you've got a child.'

Graham Archer: 'Paula's comment was really very worrying when she said that she couldn't imagine how she'd ever had time to have a job. She was a school-teacher and lived for it and enjoyed it very much. And now she's probably getting to the stage where perhaps she isn't even thinking about going back.

That's probably the worst thing that could happen. It's the child in relationship to what it might do to profession rather than any social upheavals in our social life.'

Interviewer: 'Do you think you could have children and carry on the type of career you have?'

Jane Archer: 'I've seen it done but I don't think for any one minute it would be easy . . . we've only seen it happen once in practice. It was wonderfully successful because Margaret used to go home and play with the little one, feed him, put him to bed. She was coming back to him refreshed, she was longing to see him, he was longing to see her. It was great. I couldn't see that the child was coming to any harm, in fact he was remarkably intelligent and well developed.'

For some women, however, the risk of losing control appears too great and was the initial motive behind their wish to avoid parenthood. These women had come to believe during childhood and adolescence that maternity had in some way blighted their mothers' lives: the breakdown of relationships, 'unhappiness', and the deterioration of mental and physical health were blamed on the presence of children in their parents' lives. One woman described with compassion and gratitude the heroic attempts her mother had made to provide for her family 'burdened' by a handicapped child and alcoholic husband. At 60, she was worn out, ill, yet still at work. She had been overheard saying: 'Children are a mixed blessing; they bring good things, they bring bad things'. Her daughter had articulated at an early age the desire not to have children and now, as a young woman, described her fears of being caught in a situation from which she believes there may be no escape.

Liz Finlay: 'I've got a cat, I've always had a cat and a dog, and I've got my budgie . . . animals you can leave, they're not bound to you every minute; you're not worried about what on earth they're going to turn out like. Say I had a stupid child or an ugly child, I wouldn't know what to do . . . maybe the fact it was my own I'd love it anyway, I don't know, I have a feeling the attraction wouldn't be there . . . I have a feeling probably with children I don't have that much patience; I think if they cried all day I could see myself hitting them. People say, "Oh no, you wouldn't, not your own", I could I'm sure because I know children just screaming all day, just for half an hour on end would drive me round the twist . . . I'm frightened of ending up in the house by myself because I need to be pushed to do things. I'd end up very much a cabbage, a very unhappy cabbage. I'd probably quite gladly have children if I could have a nanny; I wouldn't have the drudgery of them every day. That's very, very bad of me but I feel as if I could have a part-time job and a nanny, then I'd have as many children as we like.'

Parental responsibilities are not exclusive to women but are also central to the masculine role. Men vary in their interpretations of fatherhood. Generally recognized as their primary responsibility, however, is the provision of financial security for wife and children. This is 'identified as one of the big changes wrought by parenthood', rendering men 'more bound to their homes, their wives and their jobs' (McKee 1982: 124). Before becoming fathers they appear to 'have little idea of what fatherhood would entail and ideas of how it would affect them are extremely hazy' (Owens 1982: 78); nevertheless it is a status positively evaluated and generally accepted as an inevitable consequence of marriage. Men are expected to 'provide' their wives with children and to succour and protect the family once founded. It cannot be assumed that all men will acquiesce to this circumscription of their futures; amongst the voluntarily childless were those who shared the predominantly feminine belief that parenthood means loss of control and who during childhood and adolescence, before they had any notion of a childless future, had recognized in themselves characteristics that were incompatible with fatherhood. Alan Dexter: 'I think my views formed very much earlier than Hilary's before I had any notion that I would be able by my own efforts to create a very nice life for myself . . . For my temperament, happiness, it would be a disaster to have children'. It is widely assumed that 'men's desire for children is learned, learned in perhaps all cases as a very small child, either by identification with or envy of the mother as a childbearer or by identification with the father in his complete socially defined role as the begetter of and provider for children' (Mead 1962: 212). Men as well as women are influenced in their perceptions of parenthood by childhood experience, but again there would appear to be no direct relationship between an adequate paternal performance and a son's future reproductive aspirations. Reminiscences of some childless men suggest that in spite of fathers' expressed satisfaction with a role adequately performed, they may come to wish to avoid parental responsibilities: a wish based upon an interpretation of family life as stultifying, 'monotonous', a 'trap'. As adults, these men tend to live unconventional lives, rejecting security for experience, and, although frequently professionally qualified, eschewing conventional masculine ambitions for the sake of self-realization. They tend also to be 'truly feminist', unlike the 'neo-feminists' described by McKee, they 'espoused an egalitarian belief about the interchangeability or symmetry of men's and women's roles', and as fathers would feel obliged to 'facilitate this goal' and not expect their wives' careers to be 'sacrificed or suspended' (McKee 1982: 134–35). This belief reinforces the notion of parenthood as loss of control. The househusband may be as susceptible as the housewife to the 'cabbage syndrome' in a society that has yet to come to grips with the problems created by the often isolated nature of child-care (Dally 1982).

Men who become fathers no longer feel 'footloose, or "able to vanish to Paris" ' (McKee 1982: 133), and in this sense lose control, but loss of control may also be interpreted as reflecting the 'anarchic' nature of children. Childless men who proffered this view as having informed their desire to avoid parenthood had been only children of parents, at least one of whom had appeared to see their parental responsibilities as peripheral to their existence – included were 'elderly' parents, mothers immersed in careers, absent fathers – and had, at an early age, taken responsibility for themselves and their upbringing. They believed themselves incapable of fathering. Financial responsibility they could shoulder, but not day-to-day interaction with a small anarchic infant who, because of the fact of his or her anarchy, could not be expected to behave in a disciplined and adult manner.

Alan Dexter: 'I don't think I'd be very good at it anyway; again, without virtually devoting my life to the thing. Listening to Hilary, I'm sure you'll understand, that we both have a very ambivalent attitude to this. We both think we know, and I suspect we do know, how the ideal world would be run, how the ideal child should be brought up, but in fact, perhaps because of the knowledge of that we're not prepared to bring up the ideal child. Although in a sense we're prepared to run the ideal world but that's a different matter. You can do that without getting yourself so personally involved that your own life is intruded upon. And we are both selfish in the respect that as separate individuals, before we met each other, we were very aware of our own existence and concerned with what we wanted to do. And in getting married we were concerned that the other person would as nearly share our views on nearly all the things we'd like to do as possible, so that we fitted together and there was no question of us marrying someone who was poles apart because that would have been – have introduced stresses – doing things, wanting things, having ideas quite different to each other. Now the introduction of a child, particularly a baby, is traumatic – a third person with no concept even of the courtesy of asking before it interrupts. And it's the first seven years really that one recoils from and I basically, not mincing words, think we're too selfish to contemplate having our lives dominated by that sort of influence. At the same time in my case there is a very real recognition that this same attitude – my reaction to stupid people or awkward people or whatever – would lead me to be generally and off-the-cuff a bad father . . . it would be far too great a risk for all concerned. I think I would prove of very little use as a companion in a child's early years. I have no great sympathy with children, I don't know whether men are supposed to, but I like children in small doses. The idea of having one to oneself, on the carpet all the time, is horrifying.'

Parenthood as a complex, arduous, and demanding task

The public image of parenthood is one of plain-sailing, shared interest, romance, fulfilment, and satisfaction (Skolnick 1978). The lives of parent and child mesh in natural harmony; mothers and fathers gain in maturity and status whilst their offspring receive the physical and emotional support they require for development and growth. The existence of a mass of specialist literature and an army of child-care experts has yet to oust from prominence the belief that parenthood, particularly mother-hood, 'comes naturally' (Breen 1975; Oakley 1979). The recognition however is there that the 'natural' process can break down and that intervention in the form of education may be required. Children will learn from their parents the rudiments of family life but there is no guarantee that socialization will proceed smoothly with a socially acceptable parent as the outcome. The mother, for example, produces through her performance a powerful interpretation of what it means to be wife and mother. But, as already observed, her portrayal will not always support the dominant image; for instance, it may be so divergent that the grounding she offers in mothercraft leaves her daughter – once cognisant of what the role requires – uncertain of her own capacity to bear and rear children. Such doubts may undermine the popular belief in the 'natural' mother and parenthood becomes something of a demanding task. Ellen Vernon: 'I was not mothered as a child . . . My sister had difficulties . . . any-thing less maternal is hard to imagine except perhaps mother. I think in a sense we weren't brought up to be mothers, we don't have the right equipment.' It would appear that women are not alone in their uncertainty. Men who had been deprived of a father-figure during childhood wondered particularly about their capacity to be father to boys.

Carol Blair: 'You like children if they're nice little girls – well behaved – but if they were rampaging boys then it would have been absolutely fatal, particularly as Henry is not a sporty type . . .'
Henry Blair: 'This was something which I think was in my subconscious until I dragged it into the conscious and that was really I could not have possibly been a father to boys.'

Gaps in anticipatory socialization are recognized when alternative, even elementary interpretations of the parental role become available. These images bring to awareness and spell out what appears in others to be second nature: being different raises questions of competence. Wanting to avoid parenthood, how-ever, is not an immediate reaction. Perceiving parenthood as problematic does not tip the reproductive balance in favour of childlessness. Individuals appear to keep an open mind; men in particular with their more peripheral interest in all things to do with childbearing and childrearing, do not interpret their doubt and lack of experience as an obvious impediment to parenthood.

Doubt appears to be more likely to lead to dissension when lack of competence is interpreted as threatening a child's physical, and more significantly, mental welfare. The childless were quick to adumbrate parental responsibilities and the pitfalls of mishandling.

Cathy McCormack: 'Responsibility that you've got this life – the minute it's born, it's a human being and you don't realize the effect parents have on their children until it's too late. You might think you're bringing it up beautifully, but how do you know what the initial personality of that child is that you're moulding? You don't know whether you're doing the right thing until it's too late.'

This weight of responsibility features large in the case against parenthood. Each stage of a child's life was perceived as a minefield with every parental step likely to detonate psychological and developmental havoc. The childless find support for their views in the unequivocal statements of experts who propagate the message that 'there is a scientifically correct way to bring up children and that whatever vices their children have as adults are to be attributed, one way or another to faulty mothering' (Oakley 1982: 222). Experts may stress the role of mother but men similarly felt that 'being a parent carried with it from the outset the expectation that the father should be interested in the child's welfare and self-conscious about the business of child-rearing' (McKee 1982: 125). This does not mean that the childless believe themselves less capable than the average parent of raising 'normal', 'decent' citizens, they merely saw themselves as more responsible and more aware of possible 'failure'. A number of respondents did, however, base their rejection of parenthood on their inability or unwillingness to shoulder the responsibility. Two men, for example, described themselves as 'not good enough material' for the demands of fatherhood. They had witnessed the efforts of their parents;

experiences and observations appeared to highlight the difficulties involved.

Jim McCausland: 'My old man accepted responsibility for us, to the extent that – my God, he was determined that we were going to be, in the limits of the time, that we were going to be honest and decent and responsible citizens and he was prepared to beat the bee-jeezers out of us to make that happen and I have nothing but respect for the man . . . I never wanted a commission in the Army because I felt I wasn't a good enough piece of human material to make an officer . . . I feel the same way to some extent about kids. By God almighty, to have three or four kids and to bring them up to be decent, you know, in the Scottish sense of decent, I mean, this is a life's work. And I try to face up to a lot of responsibilities in life, but this, this is a self-inflicted responsibility . . . it's taking on a helluva lot!'

Jim McCausland was born in 1918, one of six children. His father was a miner, his mother a woman who saw children as part of life. 'I never heard any talk in my family about pregnancies, wanted or unwanted. I don't think they ever thought about it as much as that. People just got married and had kids in those days.' Through his own efforts but with the support of his 'socially and politically aware' father, he had escaped the pits; the poverty and deprivation however had left its mark and he believed children to be a drain on any but the wealthy.

Jim McCausland: 'I can remember living in a room not much bigger than this; there was my mother, my father, my older brother, me, two younger brothers, a younger sister, my mother pregnant. Just in one room. Who the hell after that would have a family! Nobody with any sense. You just don't do it, you're cutting your throat. You're beating your own head to a pulp . . . I think the worst thing that working-class people can do is to lumber themselves with kids. It holds them down and it holds the kids down.'

James Hargraves, on the other hand, had been born into a middle-class, relatively affluent family, the only child of a broken marriage.

James Hargraves: 'It's the thought that here's another individual that you've got to be responsible for 16 years and yet at the same time as being responsible for them allow them to develop as an individual. I just don't think I'm that good a person . . . I think it must be conditioned from my parents. I know they made a hash of it, I survived despite them.'

Both men doubt their capacity for parenthood, but are also aware that their reluctance contains a 'selfish' element, an unwillingness to accept a responsibility that places a child's needs above their own when it comes to allocating scarce resources, particularly time, energy, and self. Others more confident in their abilities nevertheless shared this unwillingness.

Hilary Dexter: 'I had very definite ideas on the way I was brought up and how ideally I think a child should be brought up. I was very well aware that if I wasn't prepared to spend the time and effort to do it, then I shouldn't have children . . . I don't think I could really ever have a child and then not bring it up the way I think ideally it should be brought up . . . It would involve too much effort and attention. I think it would be sacrificing things more important to me than having a child in the first place.'

This woman and others like her were ambivalent towards the parental role. She could see advantages in becoming a mother but, being unable to contemplate any compromise on the standards she believed an 'ideal childhood' requires, felt the only responsible decision was to avoid parenthood.

Parenthood obviously involves the lofty, somewhat daunting aims and responsibilities of moulding and guiding a young life, but it also involves more mundane aspects: a daily round of tasks that may appear monotonous, grubby, and unrewarding and which modern feminists have tended to stress in order to denigrate and demystify the 'Motherhood Myth'. The full-time care of babies and young children has been described as: 'Like spending all day, every day in the exclusive company of an incontinent, mental defective' (Dally 1982: 179). This hardly reflects the romance of the cereal packet image but was seen by almost half the respondents as an accurate representation and accessible justification for their decision.

Stevie Ainsworth: 'I just don't like the idea of instantly having to sort of look after them and clean up after them . . .'
Peter Ainsworth: 'neither do I, so that's important to me as well . . . I've suffered the disadvantages of other people's kids in digs, you know, noise, smell and so on.'

'Changing nappies and this sort of thing' may be off-putting but is cited more as a damning and factual statement than as a motive worthy of serious consideration. There are exceptions. Stevie Ainsworth obviously perceived the ablutionary tasks as particularly daunting:

Stevie Ainsworth: 'I don't like the idea of children filling nappies when they're in the house and the mother stretches the brat over her knee and changes its nappie, and I have to leave the room because I can't stand it.'
Peter Ainsworth: 'Just a minor thing, but we have two kittens which you despised for a couple of months, now they're on the bed.'
Stevie Ainsworth: 'Well, mainly because one of them was untrained and it used to drive me mad every time I bent down under a settee or a bed – more work to do.'
Peter Ainsworth: 'Your attitude changed radically with the cats within about a month.'
Stevie Ainsworth: 'Well, yes, I don't know what it is, I just don't like babies.'

The non-romantic image is one way of articulating a disinclination towards the parental role. Child-care may in fact symbolize 'the family', distaste for one representing distaste for the other. The daunting and for some unfamiliar prospect of catering to an infant's physical needs is one way of expressing uncertainty and communicating dissatisfaction with popular romantic imagery. Once articulated, the non-romantic image offers a partial answer to a desire to avoid parenthood that even to the individual involved may remain something of a mystery. Childhood recollections suggest that this backing away from the unfamiliar and the questionable may have underpinned the adolescent disenchantment of two men who were only children. Only children, as already observed, are disproportionately represented amongst the voluntarily childless: a possible function of their lack of opportunity to observe and witness parental activities (Veevers 1980). At the other extreme is the eldest child with more than one sibling who may be expected to take the role of surrogate parent. Veevers quotes one of her respondents as commenting: 'My father had my children for me' (Veevers 1980: 61): a sentiment echoed in this study.

Ann Knight: 'I can see myself going on forever with no children, but I cannot see myself with a child. I would have to have a complete rethink. I look at babies and I think aren't they lovely and then, for example, I was at the doctor's and there was a little boy about 18 months and he was toddling about and he looked gorgeous. He sat on the step into the doctor's surgery and left a little puddle on the step. The mother was mortified and she didn't know what to do with herself. It's all very nice but she was the one that had to rush around trying to find . . .'
Paul Knight: 'That only lasts for a couple of years.'
Ann Knight: 'Yes, I know, but I had a lot of that when I was a youngster . . . I'm the eldest sister in a family of four, two boys and two girls. As a youngster I suffered having all the responsibility and under-privileges. I had enough of my little brother sniffling everywhere, my little sister wetting her nappies and things like that to be tired of it for life.'

Distaste for catering to a child's physical needs tends to be linked to a distaste for the physical aspects of motherhood, pregnancy, and childbirth. Women need no longer fear death in childbirth but may nevertheless contemplate with trepidation the effects upon their mental and physical well-being of a condition that has become a battle-ground for factions competing for control over the reproductive process. But on the whole, childless women will describe any doubts and fears they have as 'normal'. As one woman explained: 'I'd be frightened to the extent of anybody else I've known'. Husbands tended to echo such sentiments; at times appearing even less willing to participate in a process for which they would feel responsible but which physically they could not share. They were also more forthcoming in their condemnation of pregnancy and its effect upon a female's attractiveness and sexuality. Both sexes however perceived these and similar anxieties of only minor importance.

The child as an object of 'dislike'

All adults are expected to react positively towards children (Oakley 1982; Veevers 1980); women, moreover, are expected to show a lively and maternal interest. Contrary to this view, early memories of some childless women reflect total disinterest in, open hostility towards, and little tolerance of children in general and babies in particular.

> *Marjorie Nelson:* 'Even my cousins used to get me annoyed. I always felt – I was five before my first cousin arrived – to me they were stupid and babyish. They were just ridiculous – the things they used to want to do – I had grown past that stage, I'd never really done that sort of thing anyhow. To me, to sit in the middle of a mud puddle and get covered in mud was just not on . . . They'll show you a baby and say, "Isn't she gorgeous?' To me, it's another baby and it's not gorgeous. It's a pink, wrinkled up human being'.
> *Edwina McCausland:* 'I don't particularly like babies, I've always found babies revolting.'

Although the child in Western industrialized society may be 'sacred . . . properly eliciting positive not negative emotions' (Oakley 1982: 222) the childless were not inhibited in their expression of negative feelings. The defensiveness described by Veevers in response to her question, 'Do you like children?', was not in evidence. It is possibly more acceptable in Britain than in the United States to express dislike of children in general than not to want any of your own (Veevers 1980). But like her respondents, individuals frequently made conditional statements, usually relating to the age of the child. A distinction may be drawn between babies and older children. Children may become more acceptable when capable of participation in the adult world.

> *Andrew Webster:* 'If it is possible for somebody to have a child starting at eight, when I could start to have an interest in it,

I could do things with it . . . I'd rather have a good conversation and you can't have a good conversation (with a baby).'

In this case, the eight-year-old is perceived not simply as a reactor – a dependent object demanding attention but giving little in return particularly to the 'off-stage' father – but as an actor to whom the male adult can relate and with whom he can sustain a more meaningful relationship. Andrew Webster's 'dislike' of babies is perhaps little more than an extension of the awkwardness men who are not parents experience when interacting with small children; but had nevertheless featured in his initial leanings towards childlessness. More extreme re-actions – such as revulsion and disgust – were expressed exclus-ively by women and then only towards babies; towards older children the same women appeared merely intolerant. Although varying in intensity, these reactions tend to reflect a common source: an independent and/or solitary childhood.

Edwina McCausland: 'I find babies revolting . . . I look at them and try and say something nice not to hurt the mother's feelings, but actually all the time I'm thinking, "What an ugly . . .!" . . . I was more of an only child than I should have been because between the ages of 4½ and 16½ I went to 13 different schools. So I never actually stayed anywhere to become properly integrated into any particular social group. I think because of this I missed out on some of the attitudes of my peers.'

But as the only child is not always locked within her own private world, so the child with brothers and sisters is not always prevented from withdrawing into herself.

Rosemary Hall: 'I was always happier with adults than children. In adult company I was in my element but other children, no. I would rather sit and read a book. I was a sort of loner out of four. For instance, they've all got blonde hair and they all look similar, whereas I was like my father. And people would say, "Oh, nice little girls, what's wrong with that one?" Honestly, I can remember that. I tended to be a sulky sort of kid, probably because of this. In among adults I was in my element, because out of the four of us I was the brightest and this suited me fine because I could do things that adults thought were suitable from an early age. I was really happier with adults than with children. Babies I've not really got any time for at all until they can speak. I've no time for them at all . . . I never wanted children, even when I was young, I can stand them for a wee while and then I've had enough.'

Although independence does not always presuppose solitude, the latter appears to engender a lack of familiarity with and subsequent avoidance of 'childish things' and to create a degree of autonomy that has the individual – male and female – recoiling at the thought of the small and vulnerable infant.

Susan Dobie: 'I'm a terribly independent person. I think that being an only one too helped . . . I was able to do an awful lot of things by myself and think for myself . . . Neighbours having new babies, pushing them on you, "Would you like to hold the new baby?" And I looked at it in horror . . . Toddlers weren't quite so bad, but a newly born baby really upset me, I couldn't go near it, I couldn't touch it.'

Susan Dobie did not make a pre-marital commitment to child-lessness; her disgust and general intolerance were not trans-lated into rejection of motherhood. She, like others who shared her sentiments, was conforming to the maxim, reinforced by the inevitability of the relationship between marriage and parent-hood, that states: 'When it's your own, it's different'. Women who simply 'disliked' children, succumbed – for the time being at least – to prevailing expectations. Their doubts were, however, to be resurrected and to play an important role in their eventual acceptance of a childless identity. Only where independence had been linked to unconventional family settings: handicapped sibling, marital breakdown, martyred parent, did women see their reactions to children as an obstacle to their becoming mothers. Men similarly played down the relevance of negative emotions; the implication being that mere 'dislike' is hardly justification for rejecting parenthood when the masculine role allows for the minimum of interaction between father and small infant. There were, however, exceptions; again only children

and from families where the father was either absent or conspicuously unenthusiastic about his role.

The childless as a whole appear rather intolerant of children
and childish activities. Even couples who obviously gained
considerable pleasure from their relationship with particular
children and who saw this as a significant element in their lives,
tended to enjoy their company for only a 'wee while' and were
then quite happy to 'hand them back'. There was no blanket
approval of children; both men and women were quick to proffer
examples of children who were obnoxious and badly behaved
and to question how they would react to a child who was
unattractive, unintelligent, or in some way handicapped. One
naval wife was particularly scathing:

Marjorie Nelson: 'Navy children can be real ... they've got no
  discipline. I don't see how any mother can try to be a father and
  mother to any child and still bring it up to respect people and
  things and life in general. Because we've had experiences of
  children that have been without their fathers for numerous
  lengths of time – months and years. And they're the most
  obnoxious little so-and-sos that God has ever put breath into.'

These and similar observations act to support the case against
parenthood; children may not be actively avoided but simply
being and thinking childless creates situations and routines into
which children do not 'fit'.

4

Becoming childless:
formative experiences of adulthood

Being childless implies loss, lack of fulfilment, emptiness. Whether voluntary or involuntary, it is a condition negatively defined (Mead 1962; Firestone 1972; Veevers 1980). This imagery may be assumed to provide a powerful incentive to reproductive conformity (Busfield and Paddon 1977; Blake 1979), but its one-sided simplicity fails to capture the range of alternative life-styles open to men and women, with or without children, in a society where no one set of values prevails, where privacy is a significant feature of family life, and where personal happiness and self-fulfilment are legitimate goals vying with the demands of civic duty. Involuntary childlessness may nevertheless remain a 'heavy cross to bear' (Rossi 1964); women in particular who have learnt to accept childbearing as their primary function may feel cheated by fate. Whilst the conventional feminine role is projected as woman's surest hope of happiness, the chances of her defining sterility as a blessing and building a satisfactory alternative life for herself are remote. Consequently, she may perceive her existence as futile and worthless, thus reflecting and reinforcing popular imagery. The voluntarily childless, on the other hand, are to a large extent protected from such perceptions by the intentional nature of their non-conformity; admittedly they have no children, but this does not predetermine the value of their existence.

Childlessness does not bar the individual from full participation in social life, nor do women in particular face the ostracism and avoidance experienced in other cultures (Ryan 1952). Criticism there is, but it is easily managed and far out-weighed by the perceived advantages of remaining childless. Perhaps in other marriages, in other lives, parenthood meets needs that might otherwise go unmet, but in the context of their own lives, the childless recognize neither gaps to be filled nor needs to be met by conforming to reproductive expectations. Doubt and discontent may remain, but with the decision to remain childless there is only quiet satisfaction.

Charles Quin: 'At the moment we are perfectly happy as we are. We don't feel there is anything missing or lacking.'

Evelyn Quin: 'The two of us have a full enough life . . . If you are happy with what you have and you feel that you have a complete marriage without children, why should you have children?'

The Quins believe childlessness to be in their interest. They married expecting to become parents, but had created a way of life that made children superfluous. Others making a post-marital commitment had followed a similar sequence: the situations they faced had made it possible for them to recognize the desirability and feasibility of reproductive nonconformity and to act – not always consciously – upon an emerging desire to protect the advantages of living without children.

Childlessness as comfortable routine

Much of everyday life proceeds as if by clockwork. The more settled the routine, the less susceptible it is to change. A couple who postpone conception may therefore discover that the routines they have established rule out the desirability of parenthood (Veevers 1980).

Rory MacDonald: 'There's no question that if you don't have children right away then you get into the habit of not having them around . . . I couldn't see myself now, I couldn't for the past few years . . .'

Claire MacDonald: 'It certainly would be a bit of a disruption.'

Childlessness is incorporated into their way of life; it becomes an implicit assumption informing their actions – they plan, spend, socialize, work, and relax from an increasingly childless perspective: 'When we bought our house in 1961, it had rooms for a houseful of children and when we were deciding on the function of rooms there was never a mention made as to a nursery' (Maggie Smith). Time allows for an almost imperceptible rearrangement of priorities, and although it may be possible to date the decision by referring to some alternative commitment such as 'going on the pill', accepting a university place, or changing occupation, these are little more than symbolic watersheds, points of no reproductive return heralding the acceptance of routines that have become too comfortable to disrupt. Couples may feel they did not decide to remain childless. Precautions against pregnancy are described as a response to prevailing conditions: family illness, bereavement, heavy financial responsibility.

Evelyn Quin: 'Well at the time we thought I might maybe work for a year or a couple of years and then we would have a family, but somehow things have just gone on and on and the more I think about it the less I am fussy . . . I love children basically; we are just not fussy to have children of our own. I think that the two of us have a full enough life. Maybe if our life was not so full there would be a necessity to have children. We haven't sort of said, "Right, no children, and that's that". It is just that we have gone on and we are quite happy with our various ways of life. I have had about three deaths in my family since we were married. Charles's parents don't keep good health and his father has been in hospital and we've had a lot of rushing about. My husband has not been well . . . I am less fussy about it . . . we live comfortably . . . it would be a very big change in our lives . . . the older I get the less I want to have babies.'

Accidents, they suggest, could have happened; that they have not seems to indicate – in the words of Evelyn Quin – that their childlessness 'must be meant'. 'Settled', they consider it highly unlikely they would ever decide to have children.

Rory MacDonald: 'If we sat down and decided about it now, genuinely I think I would be against it.'
Claire MacDonald: 'Yes . . . There was a time when I worked in (a town close by) . . . I'd be about 29, that I was quite keen. And then I'm 35 now . . .'

Age adds justifiable weight to a commitment motivated by the desire to protect a life-style unwittingly premissed upon a childless base; couples not only create comfortable routines but also find themselves out of touch with the reproductive timetable they see reflected in the behaviour of family and friends – their children are described as 'quite grown up'; mothers are asked, 'Would you like to start now?'.

Being 'out of touch' would also appear to provide the opportunity for couples who marry late actively to contemplate the question of parenthood. Having already thwarted convention and created independent life-styles, they are less likely to readily accept the equation marriage = parenthood.

Joan Ellison: 'I was 28, so I suppose I was older. It didn't bother me (whether I married or not) . . . I very much enjoyed being single . . . We have our way of life and children would completely alter it and of course you get older as well and you think, "Gosh, I can't start a family at this stage in life!" . . . I had been engaged before; I often think if I had got married then I probably would have had two or three children and lived in the suburbs and that would be it.'

Joan Ellison and her husband decided to remain childless: they make no attempt to excuse what was for them a deliberate choice. Other couples who admit to having made such a choice had tried but failed to become parents.

Carol Thompson: 'We were going to have children. The first two years I was going to work; I'd made up my mind I was definitely going to work two years and then – I can't remember how long it was we actually tried to avoid having children but after a while we were going to have them and nothing happened and I got fed up with all this indecision and I couldn't be bothered with it. I didn't know whether I was coming or going, going to be pregnant or not, so I went back on the pill. I can't remember how long I was on that, then we decided we'd try again.'

Interviewer: 'How long had you been married the second time?'

Carol Thompson: 'I really can't remember, maybe about four years. Maybe about two-and-a-half years avoiding having children then maybe one year where we didn't bother about contraception and then I thought I can't be bothered with this so I went back to the clinic and I was put on the pill and I can't remember, it's about four years ago (when she was 28) that we decided we were quite happy the way we were and although I love having my wee niece and nephew here I didn't really particularly want children and my husband wasn't particularly fussy . . . We don't talk about it now. I still look in prams and say, 'Oh isn't she lovely!' I think I'll always do that, but it doesn't make me definitely want to have children . . . I think who wants kids at 32 and Graham's 37. I keep thinking you're nearly 40 and it's far too old!'

The Thompsons may be unable to have children but they and others like them define their situation as voluntarily childless; they are active contraceptors and suggest that if they had really wanted children they would have sought medical help. Their decision was a simple recognition of the self-sufficient nature of a lifestyle developed over years of unsolicited freedom.

Mary Fraser: 'We were both hard up when we were first married . . . it was a conscious decision that we wouldn't have any children, I think, as most young couples do to begin with. I think like everybody else we said for two years, this magical figure, two years. It seems silly when you think about it. We didn't have any children and then once we were here and settled, then it didn't matter, it wasn't all that important whether we had any or not and, well, we didn't and that's that. So after a while we decided that we didn't see that we really needed any children . . . it was actually 1966 (when she was 30), that was when I first went on the pill . . . I'd gone up to the doctor to see about something else, it was actually me chatting away and she suggested I think about going on the pill . . . so I came back home and we thought about it and Colin said,

"Well, please yourself, it's up to you . . ." So we were going away on holiday and I said to the doctor I'd phone her up and tell her what we'd thought, so I decided yes and it was really since then . . . Quite honestly it never worried me not having any children. I suppose it must worry a lot of people but it never worried me in the very least. Probably again because of my job and being involved with children, teaching . . . when we finally decided I was very settled in my job, enjoying it, and well, all our friends had children and most of them, yes, all their children were growing up. They were all at school by this time and I suppose I must have felt a bit older – I think you've really got to be young . . . if you're having children you should have them when you're young and enjoy them. I think by the time you're a bit older your interests can't blend together really . . . I think if I had been getting neurotic about it, then we probably would have gone and seen about it, or seen if there was any possibility of us not having children or why, or perhaps even adopting a child but I didn't. So I don't suppose I must have cared all that much really.'

Mary Fraser had observed her sisters and friends as mothers and believes that she would have proved neither more nor less successful and that life would have been different but no less enjoyable; she simply likes things as they are. If however, at the age of 39, she was now to become pregnant, she would 'go mad for the first two days and then once (she'd) calmed down, (she'd) probably be thrilled to bits. But it certainly wouldn't be planned, it'd be just one of those things'. These sentiments are echoed by the other women; the two who concurred had both made substantial changes in their lives since the decision to remain childless had been made and could no longer see themselves in the maternal role. They had returned to full-time education and were now pursuing careers, actively supported by their highly educated and professional husbands. The other women either have conventionally female jobs or are housewives and like their husbands – businessmen, managers, public service employees, and skilled manual workers – had not proceeded beyond secondary education. With an average age of 38 and 35 respectively, the men and women involved in delay, whatever their social origins, appear to have been part of a generation for whom the gender roles had been clearly defined. They were aware of and had some sympathy for the issues raised by the feminist movement, but were either content or resigned to playing the roles for which they had been prepared. Childlessness had not proved to be their 'liberation' (Movius 1976); and perhaps in deference to their one major act of nonconformity, they tended to stress the normality of themselves, their way of life, their values, and their aspirations.

Charles Quin: 'I'd be out of my job (as an accountant in a bank) to-morrow, if I had the opportunity, without any shadow of a doubt. It's changed completely within the last three or four years, I enjoyed it up until then . . . it's got to the stage where it's more than flesh and blood can stand . . . I honestly don't know what I'd like to have done. I think with hindsight I'd have been much happier doing something practical, making something, being creative . . . I couldn't leave now, I don't think. We get our house-purchase; if I had to go and get a mortgage at 11 per cent, I just couldn't do it. So that when you get to my age, married with home responsibilities unless you have something lucrative to drop into, you're hooked and they know it.'

Carol Thompson: 'I wouldn't be married (if I could start again). I don't think I could get a better husband, we get on remarkably well together. We have our ups and downs like everybody else but on the whole we've got a reasonably good marriage. But I miss freedom.'

Interviewer: 'What would you like to do?'

Carol Thompson: 'To travel. I think I would be inclined to buy an old caravanette and a whole crowd of us go abroad for six months or something.'

Interviewer: 'Can't you do that now?'

Carol Thompson: 'We could still do it but you have the responsibility of having a home. You have to come back to the same humdrum existence really.'

Charles Quin and Carol Thompson appear no more likely than the average parent to drop out or kick over the traces. They and the other couples involved in delay may be described as conventional. Their decision to remain childless is a self-interested response to circumstances but one that has not entailed rejection of prevailing values; accommodation is possible since the values themselves partially justify non-conformity by stating that couples over a certain age are less eligible for parenthood and therefore less open to censure.

Childlessness as fulfilment

'Becoming and being a mother is held out as the primary feminine goal – in the 1980s, as in the 1920s or 1850s. Two women who became mothers in 1975 said:

> "It's made me feel more fulfilled. It's given me something in life. I feel that I've achieved something now. Whereas before, I mean work and everything, maybe it was the jobs I had, but I always felt like I was in a rut and was never achieving anything. But I feel as though I've done something useful . . ."
> "I feel older; you're more responsible: you've got someone to be responsible for. I suppose when you work, you just pop out for a drink lunchtime, yet I wouldn't think of doing something like that now. It's really like living in a different world."
>
> (Oakley 1979: 263)

Motherhood settles women down and provides a focus for feelings of feminine responsibility. It is fulfilling – both of the social expectation and of the personal desire' (Oakley 1982: 86). The reproductive function continues to justify woman's existence (Sullerot 1971), but no longer holds the key to fulfilment, achievement, or self-worth. Women now 'have a right, even an obligation to participate in the labor force. And not only unmarried women but wives also. And . . . even mothers' (Bernard 1975b: 118–19). With improved access to worlds outside the home, women have begun to question conventional priorities and to see marriage and motherhood as stages in the life-cycle rather than their sole occupation. They are now more able to delay pregnancy whilst gaining an education, setting up home, or beginning a career, and to limit the size of their families, providing them with greater opportunities for both work and leisure. It is just a short step from here to voluntary parenthood, to a situation where they ask 'Do *I* want to be a mother?' For a married woman to answer 'No' does not necessarily require her husband's cooperation, but for the relationship to be voluntarily childless this cooperation must be forthcoming. Husband and wife together have to accept that they, but more particularly she, have freedom of reproductive choice. Most people are likely to accept that such freedom exists whilst also believing that women who forego motherhood are in some sense abnormal or unfeminine. Couples who see childlessness as fulfilment reject this stereotype as uninformed. They were part of a generation who as adolescents and young adults during the 1960s had observed and participated in the questioning of conventional expectations and had carried the debate over into their own lives. When they took the decision to remain childless they were in their early to mid-20s and were either members of or destined for the professional middle class. Wives were career-oriented and the division of labour within marriage was based more on capability and resources such as time than on traditional gender lines.

Graham Archer: 'We are a liberated couple from most points of view.'

Jane Archer: 'You do literally share all the housework. Graham does most of the shopping.'

Graham Archer: 'I actually enjoy cooking . . . I also, within certain limits, enjoy shopping . . . There are some very nice shops on my walk back from work where I can go and potter round and get personal service and sort of pick things over. It's a very pleasant way of wandering home from work . . .'

Jane Archer: 'It happened by accident to start with because I was actually in a full-time job when we were first married and Graham was doing a post-graduate degree and just travelling down to X so many days a week so it seemed sort of natural somehow that he would do rather more in the house . . . we quite rapidly settled down into a routine where we shared everything.'

Vestiges of the traditional division of labour remain: Jane Archer, for example, had given up an interesting and well-paid job in the South of England to enable her husband to work in a Scottish university, but, on the whole, couples appear to succeed in creating interchangeable roles. One couple had experimented with role reversal.

Martin Todd: 'And then when that (university) finished I got a job after a short delay in the Forestry Commission, as a scientific assistant . . . I worked for a year in the Forestry Commission – it was a sort of probationary year. At the end of it, I said, "Oh no, it's obviously not going to be a career". So I gave that up again and then for almost two years I lived on the highly moral earnings of Lesley, just as a house-husband. And I did all the shopping and cooking, most of the housework, put shelves up and did things . . . I had a very pleasant time.'

Leslie Todd: 'He was very good at it as well.'

Martin Todd: 'Then I started getting a bit, I suppose started having scruples about this way of living . . . So I started a (legal) apprenticeship a year and a half ago . . . we always keep in the back of our mind the glowing possibility that one of us will once again be able to stop working and the other to carry the can . . . or better still, manage to find part-time jobs that will bring in enough money between us . . . We think our ideal would be a six-day week which would bring in the average salary that two people can live on. That would be nice.'

The Todds and couples like them recognize that their values and priorities may clash markedly with those of family, particularly parents, and of friends from childhood and adolescence. They see themselves in the vanguard of the movement towards freedom of reproductive choice and attribute their non-conformity to insight and knowledge gained either through lengthy education or observation and experience and to their independence, either geographical or psychological, from those to whom they are or have been attached but who do not share their unconventional views. They see no reason to question the legitimacy of their perspective; their decision they describe as a logical extension of planned parenthood. Society, they argue, allows for individual choice in the private sphere of the family and pressures individuals to seek what they seek: material well-being, occupational success, and 'freedom'. Childlessness simply facilitates the attainment of these legitimate goals.

John Blake: 'Just now our time's taken up with the house. We're doing most of that ourselves, taking out fireplaces and things . . . And we're hoping to do some planning ourselves. This is one of the things about kids, we're fairly versatile and . . . we're fairly open-minded about what we can do, a lot of people reckon because they're insurance agents or whatever, the only thing they're good at is insurance. And . . . I'm fairly nifty at woodworking and Christine's good at designing things. We'd like to open a shop making our own furniture. There's various things we'd like to do.'

Interviewer: 'Don't you think when you've done a lot of the things you want to do, like travelling, you might change your minds?'

John Blake: 'It's possible but . . .'

Christine Blake: 'I wouldn't like to think it was possible.'

John Blake: 'I think it's possible, yeah, but . . . the things like . . . when you look at things like marriage and kids and so on from outside, from just looking at society, particularly middle-class society which we've seen most of being middle-class, you just see people getting slowed down, you see their ambitions getting chopped up, their capabilities getting dulled and while it's probable that by the time I'm 35, we'll have done a fair number of things we want to do and we could possibly settle down and contemplate kids and so on. I don't think it would be necessarily good for us. I think we'd get more fulfilment from carrying on thinking of all these things . . .'.

The Todds reject the dominant image of parenthood as a source of growth and maturity (Busfield 1974; Breen 1975). For them it would be a retrograde step as they look for fulfilment through experience: experience as radical and constant change. Childlessness may also liberate at a more mundane level.

Hilary Dexter: 'I like having my own time to do what I want. I can read if I want to, go out for walks, go on holiday, all sorts of things one takes for granted . . . When Paul and Mary were up that week-end – friends of Alan's who have two children – they just came up here for a long week-end, having abandoned the children with his mother. It just came out over Sunday breakfast that that was the first Sunday morning they'd spent in bed for three-and-a-half years. I think the little things – the little freedoms I'd very much resent giving up.'

Children do not make for spontaneity. The childless are quick to recount the planning and paraphernalia involved in even minor outings.

Carol Blair: 'What puts me off, when we are away on holiday and go for a picnic or something, and I look at people with children, they've got the potty, and they've got the bottle, you know, all this, and bags with this, that, and the next thing in and . . . always having this about you, I don't know what it is. In a way I think it's a form of laziness, having to make an effort all the time, having to be pleasant and not take out your bad temper on a child . . . I might even be in the battering baby class, you know, I mean I do have a temper occasionally and . . . I would be quite frightened now to have children because I think I might lose my patience. I think I would get very irritable and . . . as far as disadvantages are concerned, having to plan anything in advance is the main disadvantage, if you're going to go out or have people round or . . .'

Henry Blair: 'Yes, because we're not planners, we tend quite often to do things on the spur of the moment.'

The childless as a whole value the freedom that accompanies their nonconformity even if they make little use of it. The stress is upon the *ability* to go out, to take exotic holidays, to move house, to emigrate whilst in reality they tend to live 'ordinary', 'unexceptional', even 'dull' lives and to identify with the reproductively conventional amongst their friends. Yet there are couples who take risks and who attribute their actions to their childlessness. Three men, for example, had left secure employment and, supported by their wives, set up small businesses or become self-employed professionals.

Bob McCormack: 'People tend to take the safe and easy, conventional way out . . . we decide that we're going to do and do it, whereas other people might decide against that because it was unconventional, it was a risk . . . it's like my going into partnership. People usually plan for years; they save up a fortune in the event of a rainy day . . . I had a fairly hefty overdraft and that was it. My bank manager nearly fainted when I went in and said, "Look, this overdraft isn't going to decrease for at least a couple of months because I've just left my job" . . . not having a family has its advantages – with a family I could never have gone into partnership. I would have had to provide security for a child because Cathy wouldn't have been able to go out to work if the thing had failed.'

Most childless women work and expect to work. Only three women were neither employed nor in full-time education – one of whom, Cathy McCormack, admitted to feeling more guilty over her 'idleness' than over her childlessness. Motherhood has been indicted as a major obstacle in women's success-fully pursuing occupational roles (Firestone 1972; Movius 1976; Oakley 1982); yet childless women, although liberated from the logistic problems of combining work and child-care, appear content to limit their ambitions to the traditional feminine occupations and to work as secretaries, shop assistants, clerks, nurses, and school teachers. Their first priority is home and husband.

Patricia Campbell: 'I have been where I am 10 years now; I find full-time nursing – it has taken too much out of me. I was never in to get Ken's meals at night and he seemed to have to come in and muck about himself. Whereas I appear to get his meal at night now . . . I think he likes it better. You can make arrangements too and you always feel more normal – not many shift-workers are women. I've thought of going to work in Marks and Spencer's or Boots', I think these would be quite nice shops to work in.'

This adherence to conventional expectations is not simply a reflection of age or lack of opportunity due to limited education; two women, still in their mid-20s when interviewed, had willingly abandoned careers upon marriage.

Ellen Kennedy: 'If in five years' time we were financially better off and I could have a part-time job, I don't think I'd hesitate . . . I don't think anyone should pretend at being a working-wife and also trying to run a house. It's not a career now; I would have jumped at the chance of promotion then which I wouldn't now.'

These conventional women, even when their earning capacity is greater than their husbands', believe that men should be the primary bread-winners. Most career women who interpreted their childlessness as an opportunity for occupational advancement, tacitly accepted, if they did not articulate this view. There was a more relaxed approach to the woman's career. It was agreed that she could make whatever decision she liked in relation to her work, the only constraints being financial. In only two cases did men have access to the same option: they and their wives appeared interchangeable. The Todds have already been described; the Hargraves were research scientists who believed in being and acting as partners with neither dominating in any sphere: 'if one of us works we both work, and preferably together'.

James Hargraves: 'There isn't a leader and a led.'
Barbara Hargraves: 'In fact there was a terrible *Which* questionnaire which came through the door.'
James Hargraves: 'They wanted to know . . . oh, it was finding out the sort of people who read *Which* and what they wanted in it. The first question was impossible to answer because it said, "Are you head of the household?" Nobody is.'
Barbara Hargraves: 'We didn't know whether to put down our rather dominant puppy. He's very aristocratic, and likes to keep us all in our place. Can you put your dog as head of the household? We couldn't decide about that question.'

Childlessness had not created this partnership; the partnership had informed the childless decision.

Two other women whose decision had been influenced by their relationships with their husbands had committed themselves to childlessness in order better to pursue their careers. They expected to gain greater fulfilment from their chosen occupations than from the maternal role about which they nevertheless remained ambivalent. Their decision was a compromise: they liked children but were already engrossed in satisfying careers. On the basis of observation and experience, they believed that only with difficulty could the two roles be successfully combined. Since they would feel obliged to put child before occupation, they preferred not to have to face that dilemma. The crucial element, however, was the husband's encouragement. Both women were convinced that if they had married more conventional men they would have conformed to reproductive expectations.

Helen Donaldson: 'One of the reasons I have some doubts about having a family is that I find it difficult to tie a family into the idea of a career, you know. I presume that if I had a family there would be a gap of a certain number of years. Well, my mother has made a very good career with that gap.'

Ian Donaldson: 'Seven years.'

Helen Donaldson: 'Seven years and she rose to be assistant headmistress within the school. So it can be done, a lot of women can do it. But I'm not sure how I would personally tie it in.'

Interviewer: 'So your career is important to you?'

Helen Donaldson: 'Very important, yes, I would say.'

Ian Donaldson: 'I am in favour of Helen having a career . . . I tend not to want her just to vegetate at home. I totally disagree with the school of thought which says that the man must be the breadwinner and the wife look after the house and so forth. I think that's an out-dated division of responsibilities. If you've got a good head on you and you're capable of doing a job and you enjoy working rather than working in the house it seems a waste both personally and from society's point of view, just to let those talents maybe be lavished on one or two children, whereas they could be lavished on a much wider number of people in the case of teaching. Well, that's my view, it's not yours . . . even though I have a secure job, either with gently or steeply rising prospects, depending on how things turn out . . . I'm still not wanting Helen to stop work at any point. I have a funny attitude towards children, I'm not sure whether I want them or not but I think I don't want children . . . at the moment I don't think I do . . . basically I just have no urge to have children. And I don't think you should have them unless you have got the urge to have them. I think the slogan, "Every child a wanted child" is a bit overdoing it because you don't know beforehand whether it will turn out to be a wanted child but in so far as I can make any judgement about it now, I don't think I really want to make the experiment.'

Helen Donaldson: 'The trouble is it's much more difficult nowadays in that you do make the decision whereas before it was . . . I would certainly not want to go back to the stage where you produced a child a year, like my grandmother did, but certainly it does make it more, if you do think about things, it does make it much more of a . . . you can turn it into what I suppose we've turned it into which is an insoluble problem, if you think about it long enough. And the thing is the longer you live with two incomes coming in and freedom and so on the less likely you are to sort of want to bring this to an end particularly when to me it would mean sort of tying me, for example, to a street like this which I hate . . . the women in the street and I have nothing in common . . . I'd hate to find I was pregnant before I could leave here. I don't particularly . . . now I can escape when it gets too much. You might be treated to next door's little tirades this afternoon, you might not, it usually gets worse as the evening goes on. She's a typical woman who cannot cope with the two children she's got, and she's pregnant with a third . . . and she drives me mad, because she brings her children up all the wrong way. Having done psychology, I suppose I know a little about how you bring up children and you certainly don't scream at them and hit them . . . the main difference between the two of us is that I get very worried about the way society's going . . .'

Interviewer: 'Do you think that really influences your decision?'

Helen Donaldson: 'I can't work that out at all, I've thought about it a tremendous amount and I just do not know. I also thought about what the position would be if I'd married someone who desperately wanted children. And then I think in that case I probably would have had children'.

Ian Donaldson: 'Yes, I think I would.'

Helen Donaldson: 'I think the fact that neither of us have been particularly keen'.

Helen Donaldson has difficulty weighing her priorities. At 27 she is unwilling to close her mind totally to motherhood.

Helen Donaldson: 'Well, I've set a date . . . my mum was 33 and 35 when she had my brother and me. Ian's mother was that old. I sort of said I must decide by 30, which gives me another three years. The job I took on as head of department I said I would do – to myself not to the authorities or anything, I would do it for a minimum of two and a maximum of four years. Well, that was when I was 26, which sort of comes to the 30 mark. And I may decide at 30 that the advantages of having a family override the disadvantages and decide at that point to have one, in which case Ian would probably agree.'

Ian Donaldson: 'Yes.'

Options can remain theoretically open until a woman reaches the menopause. Experience suggests however that the longer a couple delay, the more attached they become to the advantages the Donaldsons describe. Childless women who choose to work have difficulty visualizing themselves as full-time housewives. Enforced confinement at home through illness and redundancy had demonstrated to a number of women just how much they valued the opportunity to work.

Susan Dobie: 'I'm a secretary at the university. I don't enjoy it very much; I'm in a department where the papers are absolutely killing to type so I think if I was possibly in another department it would be better . . . I'll stick it out or go somewhere else in the meantime. I feel a bit unsettled at the moment. I usually enjoy work. Before I went down there I was at home for about seven weeks – in between jobs and I went up the wall. I thought I can't stand this. I thought at first I would work for about four or five years and then stop altogether. But that gave me a trial period and I just couldn't do it. So I can see me going on to retiral age . . . I like having something to occupy myself all day. I've got tremendous hobbies but they couldn't keep me going. I tried them when I was at home that time. After about a week or so I was really fed up. But I think it was the company I missed because there was nobody coming to see me and I had nowhere to go either . . . I don't think I'd consider giving up work, maybe part-time. I think I might enjoy that because it would give me some time at home to look after it as well.'

Working is a form of freedom: an expression of independence in both financial and physical terms. Women were particularly appreciative of their ability to make an independent contribution to the household's material well-being; couples may not be nor perceive themselves to be 'well-off' but are able to avoid or eliminate many of the worries and deprivations that appear to mar the lives of parents.

Barbara Hargraves: 'And our friends who're only just down the road, she stopped work and she's definitely going to have another baby . . . before they could just trot out, now they have to think about it every time they go out. No extra treats, not even any treats for the children. I think this is where the burden comes, where the parents are prepared to sacrifice themselves, but there isn't even the money because the cost of living has gone up so much, that they can't even calculate that. Whereas we, you know . . . it's really very selfish in a way, but we can do whatever we like.'

James Hargraves: 'We overspend from time to time but we know that there are going to be two salaries coming in.'

Barbara Hargraves: 'And we can go where we like and do what we like, eat what we like, drink what we like'.

This favourable situation was as much a consequence of the Hargraves's professional occupations and commensurate salaries as it was of their childlessness. Not all couples are or believe themselves to be so fortunate. As one young wife commented: 'We'd like to go out a lot more . . . Generally to do things we want to do but haven't got the money to do'. Childlessness also fosters realizable material ambitions.

Ann Knight: 'I'd like to be a success – to be securely well off. I'd like to be able to buy what I wanted, to go on holiday if I wanted to, to enjoy myself any night of the week, to lift myself up through buying things . . . I'd like nice things around me . . . And travelling too.'

Most couples recognize material advantage as a significant benefit that becomes integral to their case for remaining childless; only one couple, however, had made it the basis of their decision.

Diane Marshall: 'When we first got married we assumed we'd have children, sort of said, "Oh, yes, wait a year or two and then we'll have a couple of children" . . . We just assumed like everybody else. After a year we still didn't have a house or anything so it just wasn't practical, it just kept being put back and put back . . . Then when we got in a position where we'd got everything that was essential, well, we just still didn't want them and it was then we said, I don't know how it came up but it was established that neither of us wanted children at all.'

Interviewer: 'How long had you been married then?'

Graham Marshall: 'Two years . . . I always wonder whether I justify the decision not to have children by things like Meadows' publications, Forester's publications (writers on the ecological and population crises). I often wonder whether I justify the decision or if reading them led me to the decision; I'm never very sure . . . these things obviously influenced me, I don't think completely but I put a lot, well, not a lot of weight, I can . . . I sort of take the view that what was said was right but it might not be right for a couple of hundred years. At the same time I don't believe I would like to bring children into this society.'

Diane Marshall: 'The quality of life and nobody cares about anybody any more as a person. It's all material, grab, grab, grab; got to have a colour TV, got to have this. I think it's disintegrating, caring about other people and trying to help them that's sort of soft somehow. It's just being a fool if you behave like that. I just don't know where this society's going to really. This isn't my particular reason for not having children but I really think it's sick, all this violence and . . .'

Graham Marshall: 'It's true, statements like pollution controls are stricter to-day than in any other time. Well, it's true but there's far more pollution in the atmosphere than there has been at any other time. I think if you look at the figures on that, it's a good reason for you not to have children.'

Diane Marshall: 'If you did have one what sort of life would it have?'

Interviewer: 'Those aren't your reasons though, are they?'

Diane Marshall: 'No, not really. I suppose my reasons are more selfish, people say, more selfish; I just wouldn't be happy, you know. I just wouldn't like to have children, it's as simple as that . . . I wouldn't like . . . our standard of living would be just halved. And I just don't think it's worth it . . . I suppose if you had children you'd think they were marvellous and everything but . . .'

Graham Marshall: 'I think if we had an accident . . .'

Diane Marshall: 'Yes, if it happened . . .'

Graham Marshall: 'We'd do our best for a child.'

Diane Marshall: 'At first it was purely financial on my part. I didn't want to be hard up and all that, but now it's more than just financial, even if we saved enough money or say we won the Pools, I still wouldn't want them . . . I just think I'd be a rotten mother anyway because I wouldn't be satisfied myself, I wouldn't be happy . . . maybe it sounds selfish that you should only have children for what they can do for you but you still have to interact, mother and child . . . if I weren't material we probably would have had children, but I had to get so many . . . had to get a house, get this and that before I'd even consider it. Probably if we'd got married and had a family right away, we'd have been fine. If we hadn't been material we would have had them.'

Unlike Helen Donaldson, Diane Marshall is certain she will remain childless and appears to have had no difficulty making up her mind; now she 'never really thinks about it'. She has made no attempt to weigh the pros and cons of her decision; hers is a 'gut reaction' that childless means 'happy'. Parenthood can, she knows, mean 'unhappy'.

Graham Marshall: 'If you speak to somebody like Margaret across the road, they've got three young children and, I mean, she's sick to the back teeth, the thought of having the third one just about drove her up the wall, you know . . . She had it certainly but . . .'

Diane Marshall: 'She's fed up.'

Graham Marshall: 'She was really sick with the two of them, that really she . . .'

Diane Marshall: 'I mean she loves them and that and she wouldn't be without them now they're there, but she's frustrated.'

Graham Marshall: 'She wishes she'd never had them in the first place.'

Interviewer: 'I love them but . . .'
Diane Marshall: 'That's what I'd be like too.'

But Diane Marshall has chosen not to be 'unhappy' and by doing so has rejected the dominant image of desirable and inevitable motherhood and affirmed her right to choose.

Childlessness as marital harmony

In the public image marriage and parenthood are inextricably linked (Payne 1978). Marriage legitimizes the act of procreation (Malinowski 1966); procreation gives meaning to marriage (Busfield 1974). Couples are frequently asked why they married if their intention was not to become parents, and encounter the belief that their marriages are less stable than those with children and more likely to end in divorce. In response, they accept that the onus is upon them to make what they can of their relationships without this conventional safety-net of dependent child or children. They tend to stress the importance of sharing in marriage. The term 'partnership' appears frequently in their accounts. 'Tremendous amount of friendship, companionship, satisfaction, comfort, affection, security, pleasure, if you like . . . We both regard marriage as a partnership and I value that sharing aspect very much' (Charles Quin). Emphasis placed upon sharing may be interpreted as defence against trivialization: the gradual but seemingly inevitable decline into emptiness of relationships founded upon a narrow base such as a woman's beauty or a man's sexual prowess (Simmel 1964). A uni-dimensional attraction may begin to fade in the bright and persistent light of marital contact and the relationship falter unless a new focus of interest is introduced to take the edge off growing disaffection. The birth of a child may provide just such a diversion. Bob McCormack describes the process at work in the lives of his friends.

Bob McCormack: 'A lot of my friends and contacts, they have
   families. First of all they never think about it; secondly, after
   about a couple of months of marriage whether they know it
   or not they're getting on each other's nerves and the whole
   reason for two people living together seems to have dis-

appeared. So the wife has a kid that keeps her occupied and the husband can get on with his work. And it gives him certain freedom that he wouldn't normally have, like being able to go out with the boys and things like that. And though he comes home at night and handles it on his knee, it's the wife's responsibility. I don't think they consider the effect it has on their life. It's like splitting a cell suddenly; people get married as one cell and they go off as two separate people with their separate responsibilities and meet occasionally and that's it. But it's not a relationship like ours.'

Relationships without children, so the childless argue, stand or fall on their own merit. Their success is reflected in the fact that – minus the responsibilities and emotional bonds of parenthood – they simply continue.

What is or is not a successful marriage has been the subject of considerable debate and critical comment (Udry 1971; Leslie 1979). It nevertheless appears that childlessness no more than parenthood offers the key to marital 'success'. It provides no guarantee of harmony nor of lasting happiness. Kate Tennant, who enjoyed what she herself described as a very satisfying relationship, remarked, 'Marriage has been nothing like plain-sailing. I think you've got to work at being married, I really do'; and in the months following the interviews for this research three of the 44 marriages ended in separation. Elaine Morrison, who left her husband, appeared well aware of the flimsy basis to her relationship.

Elaine Morrison: 'Sometimes I think we have absolutely nothing in common . . . I like music and he doesn't. He likes stodgy food and I don't. I like parties, he doesn't. I like Beethoven, he doesn't know who he is. I like to change him, he doesn't like to change me. I think I have a sense of humour, I think that's what keeps us from completely clashing, that's what gets us together again, because we have terrific fights . . . We don't agree on little things, we only agree on big things, but little things like television programmes, closing the bread-bin, cleaning, things like that, we disagree on lots of things. I realize I'll never become like him or him like me. I think there is a lot of adjusting to do. I'll never be different, we always will have the same sort of relationship . . . I felt that I had to change to become a housewife, I didn't work for two months and I discovered that I was severely bored. I didn't like preparing lunch and supper every day, I couldn't stand the routine . . . I was bored within myself. I didn't like sleeping with someone else, I didn't like sharing, I don't like being married.'

Companionship – apart from mutual enjoyment of sexual relations – and friendship were almost non-existent within this embattled relationship. The wife, whose pre-marital commitment to childlessness had been a form of self-preservation, was unwilling to compromise in order to reach an acceptable *modus vivendi*. Elaine Morrison: 'I'm not an easy woman to live with because I don't change to suit anybody . . . I live the way I want to live and nobody is going to live my life for me at all'. Others had found compromise and the early years of marriage difficult and had faced periods of protracted bargaining.

Jacqueline Webster: 'Marriage did change our lives drastically. I didn't expect it to change our lives as it did. I suppose I was a very selfish person and I hadn't lived as close to anyone. I think in marriage you've got to give an awful lot . . . The honeymoon was fine but when you came back – living on top of one another. I would be having a bath, nobody in your family would come into the bathroom but your husband does. Small things like that. You realize how close you are to a person and how stifled you are. It takes a lot of adjusting and it took me an awful long time because as I say I'm selfish. Putting the radio on in the morning, I hate it, he likes it. There'd be blazing rows over that. It takes a bit of getting used to. I think we're only now beginning to have a good working relationship.'

Women tended to register the greater degree of dissatisfaction with the period of adjustment and frequently complained that theirs had been the more radical change.

Pauline Adams: 'I can remember coming back from my honeymoon, we were sitting in the plane and I thought, "I wonder how I'll be managing this time next year?" I don't think a man's life changes very much, do you? They just change from one woman running their life to another . . . Bob doesn't do any housework . . . Sometimes I mind but you just accept it. Once you're married, that's it, you've just got to get on with it haven't you?'

Relationships least likely to engender such comment were those of couples who from the outset had rejected conventional interpretations of masculine and feminine roles and who saw marriage primarily as a form of friendship; sharing thoughts, hopes, and fears, seeing the world, its inhabitants, and its happenings from a similar perspective. There was, however, a category of unconventional couples whose striving for self-fulfilment and independence had found and continued to find expression in conflict.

Jim McCausland: 'We get along alright . . . we don't have quarrels, we have fights . . . it's a running battle. A lot of truces in it and we have a lot of fun together and we have enough common ground to meet in and so on . . . As two people who live together, see a helluva lot of each other, have sex together, have fights together, eat together, we fish together and do a whole lot of things together, by and large we get on quite well.'

Jim McCausland's assessment of his marriage is echoed in the accounts of other men and women; marriage is admittedly demanding, but given the problems they have or might have faced, couples on the whole feel a certain sense of achievement. Their marriages have 'worked' and appear to compare favourably with those of friends and acquaintances (Veevers 1980).

Jim McCausland: 'Certainly all working-class people and this is even more true of a few middle-class people I know, Christ, they're leading lives of quiet desperation, but I don't know what type of marriage we have. We get along alright . . .'
Edwina McCausland: 'There aren't very many happy marriages amongst our friends, are there? And then we usually say we're glad we're us and we've got our relationship rather than the one that is just breaking up . . . I don't think we think whether or not we have a good relationship, a good marriage, we just have what we have, presumably we like it because we're still together.'

Childless couples are divided on the question of children and marriage. They accept that the birth of a child – particularly the first – adds a new dimension to marital interaction but reject the convention which states that this will be positive, making possible greater harmony of interest, unity, and affection, and offer an alternative interpretation of coalition, realignment, and increasing distance. They cite their observations and experiences of family life as evidence; but when asked to evaluate the effect of a child upon their own relationships they are less assertive, less dogmatic. Changes might be dramatic but not always destructive. The determining factor is the nature of the relationship involved. There is no one childless marriage: they range from the embattled to the vital and total as described by Cuber and Haroff (1963). These marriages approximate to the romantic ideal: in vital relationships partners are generous with themselves and with their time. They obviously enjoy being together. Enjoyment is not their only reward, the friendship they establish offers support, encouragement, and the security that comes from knowing that united in spirit they face the world (Berger and Kellner 1970). It is a unity that recognizes, respects, but is able to transcend, conventional definitions of male and female. The result is a togetherness that couples perceive as reaching both practical and psychological limits.

Sandra O'Neill: 'We shoot and fish together . . . I decide what's for tea! It's very difficult because with us not having children, I don't know, but I find that I have a very much closer relationship with my husband than a lot of people I know with children. I mean things like making tea, I organize that. I wash and do all those sort of things, but we do the garden together and things like that and decide . . . Jimmy doesn't go out and say, "I'm having that, that and that", he asks me first and we decide together. And we sort of paint the house together and do bits and pieces. We do so much together that it's very difficult to say what I do and what he does.'

Although Sandra O'Neill works and would not want to be 'tied' to the home, marriage and being a good wife remain her central concern. She would certainly share the opinions of Rosemary Hall, 'I like what I'm doing (bank clerk). I don't want a lot of pressure because if there's too much pressure at your work then your home life suffers and I'm not really in favour of that'. Men are also actively concerned in sustaining and building upon the strengths of their vital relationships; weaknesses, when identified, are subjected to painful, yet sympathetic, scrutiny.

Sandra O'Neill: 'Again at one time I was always saying that I can't do things, you know, and you said, "You'll have to do it because I won't be there". I more or less had to be pushed to do things. And it sort of went against the grain a bit because I thought he was being unkind. Then I discovered six months later that he wasn't being unkind, it was all for my own good . . . I would say that Jimmy and I could discuss anything from the Bible to bottoms, which we could, couldn't we, Jimmy? We could talk about anything. I mean there again . . . the sort of problems I had and if I didn't talk to Jimmy about them I couldn't talk to anybody else. And that's what I want, I don't want to talk to anybody else about a problem I have, when I've got a husband sitting at home, I can talk to my husband.'

The O'Neills' enthusiasm and intention never to stop learning about and being alive to one another's needs were indicative of vital marriages, but like other couples they recognized that too much involvement might suffocate and made conscious efforts to develop separate interests, cultivate personal friends, and 'do things alone'.

Jimmy O'Neill: 'We accept the fact that we can't work together 24 hours a day, she has her own job. And it works very well. We understand the need for that actually as well.'
Sandra O'Neill: 'Too close contact just wouldn't work.'
Jimmy O'Neill: 'There are times when I go off to Ireland for a week or more and she might go off and stay with a friend for a few days.'
Sandra O'Neill: 'Which we both enjoy because I look forward to coming back.'

Vital relationships appear loving, open, and generous: an environment public imagery suggests is ideal for parenthood and which most couples believe would not have been damaged if they had decided to have children.

Mary Fraser: 'It is very difficult to say whether it would have been better or worse had we had children . . . I would have hoped that had we had children we could have enjoyed doing things with them. This doesn't always work out with couples . . . if you do have children you just have to recognize that you cannot do certain things until the child is older. Mind you, there's not a lot you have to curtail because if you really enjoy your children you can get the two together quite well . . . children are not all that fragile, you can cart them about most places.'

Interviewer: 'Do you think a child would come between you?'

Mary Fraser: 'I don't think so. I think it depends on the child's nature too. I would have hoped that if we'd a child or children that they would have enjoyed coming out on the hills with us and seeing places with us, reading, music, this sort of thing. And I think probably they would have.'

Not all couples were as confident as Mary Fraser; two had in fact taken the decision to remain childless to protect their vital relationships in which one partner was so emotionally dependent upon the other that a child's presence would have been resented.

Mary Johnson: 'I must feel wanted, that's part of my make-up. I have to feel wanted and needed . . . I can be wanted and needed by Douglas. I can force him to want me.'

Douglas Johnson: 'I don't think children would add any security.'

Mary Johnson: 'I think less because I'd get less of his attention . . . I definitely need his attention.'

Douglas Johnson had adapted to his wife's desire to keep their marriage relatively closed yet neither partner believed in total immersion. Mary Johnson cultivated her own interests outside the home; she simply refused to share her husband's scarce emotional resources. Theirs was not a total relationship and like most childless couples they believed that too much together-ness might prove claustrophobic. The three couples who had achieved 'oneness' did not feel trapped nor eager for fresh air but were digging themselves deeper and deeper into marriages that gave them cause for eloquent description,

Barbara Hargraves: 'We just went together so well that we don't know whether sometimes we are two sets of people or whether we're one head with two bodies . . . we're really our best friend, completely complete, the two of us.'

Although the Hargraves's decision had not been based on a desire to protect their relationship, they recognized that it was now central to their commitment, and had eclipsed all prior considerations. Martin Todd expressed similar sentiments:

'I think the situation now is that we've built up a kind of self-sufficient life for ourselves which I enjoy very much . . . I would resent, I think, an intrusion into this now. I think that's the largest factor . . . we have little cones of silence that we enjoy, enjoy building around us and children literally take you out of yourself and I think that we've both discovered that we're very happy with ourselves in a sense that we are both . . . are a self, I think of us as an individual almost, as a kind of individual organism, sharing very much the same kind of life.'

But for most couples 'oneness' is not an issue. Of more general concern is a relationship's satisfying tempo, the predictable way of things summed up in the statement, 'We get on fine as it is'. Relationships described in such modest terms run on an even keel: an area of compatibility created over years of compromise or initial agreement. Husband and wife may be friends who build a haven where they can be themselves (Berger and Kellner 1970). They may also share decisions and responsibilities within the home, but there is no obvious striving towards an egalitarian division of labour nor towards constant companionship; who does what depends more upon weight of external commitments, recognized competence, and personal preference. The only proviso is that the compromise division must be seen to be fair.

The fairness and security of this type of relationship act as a perfect foil for satisfying and demanding careers. Professional couples involved in even keel marriages believed that independence and compatibility were the recipe for a stress-free and supportive home-life. The Dexters, both career civil servants, had contemplated no other form of marriage.

Alan Dexter: 'I think both of us were and still are very independent people. But we just decided it was very much better being together than otherwise . . . we are both selfish in the respect that as separate individuals before we met each other we were very aware of our own existence and concerned that the other person would as nearly share our views on nearly all the things we'd like to do as possible, so that we fitted together. There was no question of us marrying someone who was poles apart because that would have introduced stresses – doing things, wanting things, having ideas quite outside . . .'

Commitment to childlessness was one of the areas of Alan Dexter's life he required his future wife to share and their relationship was based upon the premise there would be no children. They had created a haven which would be destroyed unless the birth of a child was fused into their marriage in such a way that the basic criteria of independence and compatibility remained intact.

Hilary Dexter: 'You would expect me to look after it and yet I think you would be mildly, if not strongly, jealous of the attention which I'd inevitably have to give the child.'
Alan Dexter: 'I fear so, yes.'
Hilary Dexter: 'I think it would grossly interfere with our relationship unless it was a completely shared responsibility.'
Alan Dexter: 'It might work out later once . . . and then only if the child was such that . . .'
Hilary Dexter: 'And the damage to our relationship would have been done.'

Couples who, unlike the Dexters, had married expecting to become parents admitted the possibility of initial strain but recognized no lasting threat to the fairness and security that characterized their relationships.

There were other even keel relationships based less on friendship and more on companionship where husband and wife shared certain activities: hobbies, decisions, responsibilities, tasks, but to a lesser extent a common reality. Marriage they described as 'a pleasant place to be'. According to Geoff Young, 'I don't honestly think I could say I'd been unhappy or that I've been head-over-heels having a great time. It's perfectly normal'; his wife's response, 'It's a nice way to live'. Couples involved in this type of relationship tended to be conventional in their interpretation of the sex roles. Friendship is superficial and companionship may be restricted to mainly leisure-time activities. Three women had decided to remain childless to prevent further segregation and the strain this would have placed on their relationships.

Joan Ellison: 'We can just put our coats on and go out . . . I mean if Jack wanted to go out and he wanted me to come with him and I said, "What about the kids? I can't get a baby-sitter", well, that is how many men go out on their own all the time, this is the reason the women are stuck at home with the kids and I don't see why that should be the case . . . we can just go where we like, when we like.'

Wives like Joan Ellison had accepted their husbands' definition of their role, had limited their ambitions to work not careers, and expended most of their enthusiasm on their home-making and social activities. Husbands were the dominant partners: a feature of marriage not always appreciated by wives who nevertheless described themselves as 'happy enough'; they had not expected marriage to be otherwise.

Maggie Smith: 'I didn't have any romantic notions that everything would be marvellous with me standing there in a frilly apron in a dream of a house. I wasn't pessimistic but almost. I'm terribly realistic about things. I expected marriage wouldn't change your world into bliss . . . Neither of us are unreasonable. If he gets kept late at the office I don't think that's a reason to go off the deep-end, if the dinner's been ruined, this sort of thing. And he doesn't expect me to be there with the meal ready on the dot, never has.'

Relationships 'jog along'. Sensible and happy the arrangement may be, but lacking in zest and vitality. This is not to suggest a disinterest in sexual activities; sexual relations are engaged in with varying degrees of enjoyment by both men and women. What is absent is any sign of unbridled delight.

Childlessness does not rule out the viability of erotico-romantic relationships.

Bob McCormack: 'That (emotional and physical satisfaction) is our relationship. We didn't get married so that we could sit there at night, me reading *War and Peace* and Cathy, Beckett and swapping intellectual anecdotes. That's it, we enjoyed each other, our company and our bodies. It's not a marriage of minds or anything like that, like Lord and Lady Longford, Lord Longford said his best friend was his wife. Cathy would be grossly insulted if I called her my best friend.'

Cathy McCormack: 'It makes me feel like a dog!'

Within this type of relationship men and women do not aspire to friendship, preferring to base their relationships upon a shared sexuality and a level of companionship that augments this more physical contact. It is as lovers and not as marriage partners that they interact.

Kate Tennant: 'I'm very happy with the way things have turned out. After 10½ years I still fancy him . . . my marriage is the way I like it at the moment. I have a great sex life in my marriage, I think it's one of the most important bits of our marriage. We have a gorgeous sexy marriage.'

Where a wife is a lover before she is companion or friend, where marriage is first and foremost a sexual relationship, motherhood, so couples argue, would undermine, if not totally destroy the relationship's sensual and highly pleasurable core by lowering the female's level of involvement and by reducing her sexual appeal.

Paul Lind: 'I'm rather scared of what it might do to our relationship, not in the sense that my nose would be put out, but you hear all sorts of things about women's sort of sexual thing . . . decreasing or altering . . . a woman who has had a child is different from a woman who hasn't . . . they have a totally different approach to you once they get used to the idea of motherhood . . . When she comes out of the hospital with her little bundle of joy, it's not the same Kim that I know . . . she'll still feel the same way about me in a way but in another way not really'.

The erotico-romantic relationship appears to be more than a passing phase in the first flash of passion; of the four couples in the category, two had already survived their 10th anniversary. Relationship and childless commitment grow together but so also does the realization that marriage based upon sexual attraction may be subject to trivialization. As in vital relationships, couples make a conscious effort to develop separate interests and to live independent existences.

Jeannie Maxwell: 'I have a husband whom I adore and after 11 years I still adore . . . I'm a very free person, it's not the sort of relationship that makes demands on each other. Simon also has a reasonably separate life. We can be two very separate people but we are also very much a unit. We do care very much about each other . . . I want to make things happy for him . . . Our sex life to us is marvellous. I'm always terribly happy with my husband.'

It is perhaps interesting to note that Jeannie Maxwell and the other women who accepted the erotic image had all experienced early independence and a childhood that lacked a mother-figure. The wife as lover offers a continuation of a prized independence but with a welcome security as additional bonus: a husband but not the trappings of home and family.

The childless as a whole reject the popular image of the family as a natural and harmonious triangle with its sides held firmly in place by children at the apex. They recognize their interpretation distorts popular imagery and therefore look for justification to add weight to a case based upon their own satisfactory and happy marital experience. Conventional marriages are an obvious target.

Rosemary Hall: 'Mothers tend to put the children first . . . I've seen my sisters. They tend to have arguments and I think it would be avoided if there weren't any children. The children cause these arguments to a certain extent.'

Similar observations were frequently made. Even when a relationship was described as working well, it was usually found wanting in some important respect. This critical process reinforces the wisdom of the decision to remain childless.

Stevie Ainsworth: 'We've got a couple of friends who are quite exceptional in a way, they still have their private lives . . . But I wouldn't like to be them, they cope incredibly well having two children . . . but I don't think I could do that because . . . I like to spend time with you . . . And go out with you, not separately like them.'

Triadic experiences are also recounted.

Helen Donaldson: 'We have been so very close, we know exactly what each other's reactions will be to things and so on, you could imagine that . . . any time there has been a third person connected to us, there has tended to be a difficulty. David isn't now . . . he and I actively didn't like each other for a very long time.'

Cathy McCormack: 'We had a trial with a kitten – this is what really did it. We sent the kitten back after a week. It was sad but . . .'

Anecdotes, observations, experiences provide an objective backdrop to the childless interpretation of parenthood as a source of marital difficulties but subjectively are accorded only minor significance when compared with the living proof of their own satisfying, and at times rewarding, relationships.

Childlessness as condition for marriage

Marriage is a merging of biographies that requires a degree of compromise if security and support are to be the outcome (Berger and Kellner 1970). Individuals who have made a premarital commitment to childlessness must decide whether to

reverse their decision when faced with a reproductively conventional prospective marriage partner or to try and persuade the
other to accept their position. Four couples had gone through
this experience, with the more conventional partner accepting
childlessness as a condition for marriage. Conversion may go no
further or, as in Robert Nelson's case, lead to total commitment:

Marjorie Nelson: 'He knew before I married how I wouldn't have
   any children.'
Robert Nelson: 'I originally wanted children or at least I thought
   I wanted children and I was hoping that eventually Marjorie
   might change her mind. Well, I say I was hoping, it was in the
   back of my mind. But over the years, I don't know. I don't want
   children now either and I can't conceive of any situation where
   I might want them. I think possibly at the time it was a slightly
   immature wish that I suppose children would give me that bit
   of maturity. There are various reasons one has for having
   children. I've gone past that stage and having done it without
   children, I don't really want the encumbrance – to me children
   now would be an encumbrance: an unnecessary, unwanted
   encumbrance.'
Interviewer: 'What was your reaction to Marjorie's decision?'
Robert Nelson: 'We weren't even courting when we were discussing it. We were just friends then. I think I believed her. As I
   say, at the time, I had the thought in mind that she'll change
   once she's married and settled down, she'll change. But then
   again we got married, but we've never settled down till now.
   I think I just liked the idea of having children, I didn't really
   want children if you know what I mean . . . It would be the
   inconvenience. The Navy makes you very, very self-sufficient.
   You rely on each other to a certain degree but you look after
   yourself completely. There's no one there to do your washing
   for you, you do it all yourself. And you tend to look on people
   who rely on you as being – it's not the Navy's way of doing
   things. It's the thing – the thing I can do with a dog that I
   can never do with a child. I've said I do stick to routine.
   Occasionally I come in from work, the dog and I have a set
   routine; it gets fed and I take it out for a walk. I sometimes just
   can't be bloody bothered to take it out for a walk. So I kick it out
   of the door quite literally. And I go out quarter of an hour later

and bring her in. She's quite happy to do that. When I'm like that she'll come in, curl up in the corner of the settee; she'll disappear. If I'm in a playful mood, she'll play. With a child you can't do that, the child makes its demands on you. Whereas I make the demands on the dog. In fact a child is the master. Very sorry, no one's my master not even in the Navy. It's that and obviously the money as well. The expense of a child would greatly – make inroads into my life as far as money goes. I'm selfish.'

A life without children provides couples with more room to manoeuvre, whatever their situation and intentions. Their relative freedom symbolizes their selfishness: a failure to accept adult responsibilities. In recent years, however, attention paid to problems of 'global survival', and more specifically but relatedly to the wider implications of individual reproductive choices, has provided a rationale for remaining childless that presents those who make this commitment in a more responsible light.

Childlessness as moral responsibility

Parenthood is a social responsibility, but parents also have a moral responsibility towards their children. They are expected to provide for, shelter, and protect them, and prepare them for a responsible adulthood. Not everyone feels equipped for this task, not solely because of their own 'inadequacies' but also because of adverse social conditions: economic uncertainty, political and social unrest. Amongst the voluntarily childless were men and women of varying ages and backgrounds who saw the parental role as particularly onerous in today's world and who questioned the morality of bringing a child into so uncertain a situation.

Charles Quin: 'I don't know if this country as it is now is necessarily a good place to bring children into. It frightens me, the thought of the future. Twenty years hence is it going to be a world for a child to live in or to grow up in? It frightens me to see the general trend of things . . . I think if we had a child I would be very considerably worried about its future at the moment. I mean obviously things may improve within a few year's time, you can't tell. Trends seem to be away from it at the moment with increasing violence, and crime and lack of respect for law and order, hijacking, inflation, you name it, we've got it. It would worry me if I were a parent just now quite apart from the basic things like education . . . I would be worried for the child . . . It's another factor to consider. I don't think that in itself would be sufficient to influence us if we decided particularly that we wanted a family all else being equal.'

Ken Campbell expressed a widely held opinion when he said, 'I don't think I'd thank anybody for bringing me into this world as it is now and how it's going to be'; such pessimism was seen as a burden children should not be asked to share.

Martin Todd: 'One factor that I don't want to make too much of is that neither of us are very happy in the world which is why we do tend to create our own bubble of solitude. We both get very upset by events which force themselves upon us and I think I would always think twice about bringing a child into the kind of future that looks as though it's going to befall the human race . . . we couldn't bring them up in an optimistic way, because we're not optimistic. And I think the troubles of the world would sit very heavily on them as they have on us in some ways.'

As Martin Todd admits, these views had not informed his commitment to childlessness but had become more salient in response to prevailing social conditions and would be a consideration in any future deliberations. Others believed their pessimism was irrelevant to their decision or any possible change of mind but acted as a justification since their more 'selfish' motives were socially suspect. There was one exception:

Betty Hamilton: 'I think before you have children you have to have a belief in something to pass on to your child, to give it some reason for living. I don't think I could offer a child enough, certainly not at the moment . . . I don't think it's a particularly good world for them to be in. I can't see that perhaps by the time my children are my age that there will be very much to make it worth living. At the moment I have little or nothing to give to a child and society certainly has nothing worth giving to anyone.'

This is a deeply considered and highly personal commitment to childlessness that reflects Betty Hamilton's attempts to come to terms with herself in the world. She had not succeeded in doing so, and refused to take responsibility for bringing an innocent child into a similar anomic situation. Adding to her concern were problems of physical survival: over-population, pollution, food-shortages, natural resource depletion.

Childlessness as social responsibility

The population problem and related issues provide the childless with a semi-respectable front; amongst intellectuals in particular it appears to be a sign of commendable restraint and personal sacrifice (Veevers 1980). Adherence to this meaning, however, is not always an act of self-defence. There were those who believed that ill-considered parenthood is socially irresponsible and that their own decision could be perceived in altruistic terms, although it is in fact based upon personal motives, rather than any consideration of wider social interests.

Rory McDonald: 'It may be hindsight but I'm absolutely appalled at this business of seeing some smiling couple who've been married a hundred years and they've got 10 children, and sort of a 130 grandchildren, and of course their descendants number 5,336. If we all did this we'd never be anywhere. And yet people don't seem to think this way, not when they're having children. That's not any decision we've made but it's a fairly strong view I have.'

Social responsibility is a secondary consideration: a relevant fact; if couples were to contemplate children they would attempt to limit their number but would not deny themselves the experience for the good of the global community. Once commit-ted to childlessness, couples of all ages are jealous of their right to choose. Rosemary Hall expressed a general opinion when she said, 'I'll argue with anybody who says everybody must have children. I just say, "No, no, no one must have them at all". If you want them by all means have them. If I ever did have a family it wouldn't be because I decided that everybody else was right and I was wrong. It would be because I felt I wanted a family, felt I could sensibly have a family and give a good life to a child. Not because everybody else has children and I haven't'. These sentiments appear to support the perspective that sees voluntary childlessness as a further demonstration of 'the increasing centrality of individual goal attainment, that is, the individual's right and freedom of defining both goals and the means of achieving them' (Lesthaeghe 1983: 429). A close look at Rosemary Hall's biography, however, indicates that her commitment to childlessness was not based on rational calculation but was a response to childhood experience. 'I never wanted children, even when I was young . . .' Cost-benefit analysis came later as she attempted to justify her nonconformity; her rejection of the inevitability of parenthood is a demand for freedom of reproductive choice. In the mid-1970s in Scotland this freedom did not exist. The voluntarily childless defined themselves as deviant although they believed the label unjustified given the extent to which pursuit of personal goals was an acceptable motive for conformity to reproductive expectations. The confrontation between those who conform and those who deviate creates problems for both sides. Parents, seeking to condemn or persuade the childless of their folly, face the difficulty of articulating assumptions and motives that may have previously lain dormant, whilst the childless, made aware of prevailing imagery, must find a way of counteracting with an interpretation of their own and of parental behaviour that defends their unconventional position.

5

Parenthood:
public relations and the childless

If there is a conspiracy to persuade the childless to become parents (Waller and Hill 1951), it would appear to be their conforming peers who are the most persistent in their attempts at recruitment. Persuasion takes the form of a public relations exercise that extols the virtues of parenthood whilst disparaging the childless alternative. The childless dodge, parry, face up to, and even contradict, but rarely succumb to this flow of publicity working to wear down their reluctance to play the game. If, however, they manage to evade the message so clearly relayed and to recognize the contradictions and anomalies between parental word and deed, they may still have to confront and elude the skirmishing tactics of – amongst others – parents, colleagues, acquaintances, strangers, and the mass media.

Joan Ellison: 'We were sitting one night watching the television and there was a remark made about, "You're no man, what have you got to show for it?" You know, no children for this man to have proved he was a man. We just sat and looked at each other and said, "Gosh, it comes at you from all angles". Any young couple sitting watching that perhaps they would be intelligent enough to see through it, but everybody isn't intelligent enough to realize that this is pressure, because that's what it is really.'

The childless become attuned to registering these cues. Their sensitivity, linked to a sometimes constant stream of opinion and observation, provides them with an outsider's insight into the mechanics and motives of parenthood. The information they receive is in turn used to construct an interpretation of fertility behaviour supportive of their childless commitment.

The mechanics: becoming a parent

The childless describe most people as taking parenthood for granted.

Cathy McCormack: 'I've spoken to lots of newly married wives – friends – and say, "Are you going to have children?" And they say, "I'm on the pill just now, I've thought about it, I don't really want them *but . . .*", and you say, "Why but?" And they say, "Everybody has children".'

Because having children is 'what everybody else does', it is the normal thing to do; and because it is normal, it carries the weight of inevitability.

Ken Campbell: 'A lot of them just have babies because . . .'
Patricia Campbell: 'It's the thing to be done.'
Ken Campbell: 'They feel out of it if they haven't got one to push along the road.'
Patricia Campbell: 'I think it just happens; they take it for granted.'

The normality and inevitability of parenthood implies that 'doing what everybody else does' is the right thing to do; the push to imitate and conform is therefore reinforced by moral pressure. Parenthood becomes a duty. Ellen Kennedy: 'I'm sure it's just a matter of society again. One expects you to have children so a lot just automatically have children without really thinking of it . . . you feel you should have children'. Ellen Kennedy had herself experienced considerable pressure to conform, but remained adamant in her belief that there was freedom of reproductive choice. The childless as a whole condemn blind acceptance of parenthood's inevitability. Some go on to explain their own ability to sidetrack normality as a consequence of their more favourable circumstances. Age, status, geographical and social mobility, and social isolation are frequently mentioned as factors that might differentiate them from those unfortunately press-ganged into parenthood.

James Hargraves: 'I think there is a lot more pressure on a woman. All the advertising, the media are geared to the image of woman as mother. And I think there is so much pressure that a woman may, must in certain circumstances feel incomplete without children.'

Barbara Hargraves: 'I think here actually the atmosphere isn't all that bad. John . . . was saying that his wife was a teacher and wasn't sure whether she particularly wanted children but she kept seeing colleagues leaving term after term and having children. It was the accepted thing, whereas there are a lot of women here who work, who don't have children, who are perfectly happy . . . I think where the pressure isn't definitely upon you and where it isn't considered the norm to trot around having children then you consider yourself very much more carefully what it is *you* want, and what *you* should be doing in the circumstances.'

The implication being that if other women found themselves in similar situations they would take the same decision, or at least consider childlessness a viable alternative. This interpretation allows the childless to protect and justify their own commitment whilst respecting the integrity of those who conform (Lyman and Scott 1968). A less charitable view counterattacks by denigrating parents; to neutralize criticism individuals may express contempt at the majority's blind conformity (Matza and Sykes 1957; Veevers 1980).

Susan Dobie: 'I think they are naïve, they obviously haven't thought about it (parenthood) properly, gone into the ins and outs of it, they've just been geared to the one idea. I think I'm perhaps superior because I've thought it all out. I realized there was a choice whereas they haven't, they've gone into it without thinking.'

Even Susan Dobie had to admit that if parenthood is taken for granted so also is the need to plan. Parents try to limit their families: a concession sometimes hastily qualified by reference to the lack of success couples have particularly when it comes to timing. Claire MacDonald commented: 'A lot of my friends have had them not when they really meant to have them, they wanted to wait till they were more settled but an accident came along'. Accidents do not always become unwanted births. The childless describe most of their friends as happy with the number of children they have and their families, at least in relation to size, as planned. They nevertheless continue to see as culpable the unthinking, haphazard, and at times accidental way in which couples take upon themselves the onerous duties and responsibilities of parenthood.

Claire MacDonald: 'All our friends had three or four babies right away. And you were shocked, well, not shocked but you thought it was awful ... you used to get upset about this non-thinking of theirs or something ...'

Rory MacDonald: 'Well, you found almost inevitably that they hadn't really planned to have them. And I thought it was just curious, I couldn't understand it. They always said, "Oh, gracious, it's terrible and we can't afford it and we're struggling to do this". The attitude I took then and still take is what the devil is the point in having children unless you're someone who likes children genuinely *per se'*.

These and similar observations reject parenthood's public image as distorted and misleading. Once the spell of inevitability is broken, images of the future for husband and wife with or without children ramify and with them, for those yet to decide, the problem of choice; making a decision may become an almost impossible task. Individuals may feel threatened by lack of direction, by the void in which they find themselves. Feelings of being adrift may go some way towards explaining the social isolation and distance experienced by some individuals during the initial stages of their childless careers and why the uncertainty may linger in the fears expressed by some women as to how they will react once they have reached the menopause and the choice of motherhood is closed. Whatever the fears and however intense the dilemma, being aware of and being able to make a choice are perceived as infinitely preferable to the consequences of ill-considered parenthood.

The motives: why be a parent?

The impression that parenthood is an ill-considered step deepens as the childless become aware of what appear to them to be the 'out-dated', 'trivial', 'morally reprehensible', but socially acceptable motives put to them by those involved in reproductive recruitment.

PARENTHOOD AS THE KEY TO MEANINGFUL MARRIAGE

That marriage and parenthood are intimately related is reflected in a question frequently asked of the voluntarily childless: 'Why did you get married if you didn't want children?' Marriage, as Malinowski suggested, tends to legitimize reproduction and not the simple and in itself innocuous act of copulation.

Sheila Kidd: 'Sometimes I think it's a very sort of selfish attitude – to get married if you're not going to have children because people keep getting at you, "Why did you get married?" . . . I was fed up one day at work and I happened to say I was fed up and this woman said, "Oh, never mind, this time next year you'll be having your first one". And I said "Oh, never!" And, "Oh", she said, "Why on earth did you ever get married!" '

The childless are surprised, insulted, and sometimes angered by the implications behind these comments.

Allan Oliver: 'I tell them to mind their own bloody business. There's more in life than just having kids. It never entered my head that I was marrying Brenda just so we can have a family . . . I'm not marrying Brenda as a breeding-machine.'

The childless are not unusual when they deny the importance of parenthood for their decision to marry. Most men and women place little emphasis on the parental qualities of a prospective mate (Blood 1962). Before marriage the question of children may be given scant consideration, parenthood being a hazy commitment to be realized at some future time. Marriage, however is not static; as a series of stages informed by a cultural timetable it changes both focus and rationale. People can marry for love or companionship – both highly acceptable motives – what is not acceptable is that the unit maintain its exclusivity indefinitely. Marriage commits couples to parenthood, to 'the family'; if they fail to realize this commitment their marriage appears meaningless to observers whose awareness of the normality of the marriage/parenthood sequence is heightened by the incompleteness of a family consisting solely of husband and wife. The childless reject as limiting and outdated this notion of a natural unit made up of mother, father, and child, preferring to see each marriage as a personal statement the meaning of which rests with the two people involved and not with an oblivious conformity to public imagery.

Maggie Smith: 'In some cases, obviously not always, people think the family should be a unit. There should be mum, dad and children . . . I don't think not having children is right for everybody, it might be very wrong for a lot of people. People like my mother for whom a marriage was children.'

Maggie Smith had never been asked to justify her decision to marry and remain childless but was no less aware of the widespread acceptance of the assumption linking marital and parental roles or of the belief in a child's value as marital insurance.

PARENTHOOD AS MARITAL INSURANCE

Although available evidence suggests children may offer little protection against marital breakdown (Gibson 1980), the childless believe that people around them see their marriages as suspect because they have no children. Remarks are rarely made directly but from indirect sources such as the media the message linking parenthood to marital success filters through. They simply refuse to accept this blanket assessment, sometimes only to reverse it, frequently to replace it with an open verdict. Charles Quin said: 'I think you can have a perfectly happy marriage and relationship without children. I don't think it's essential at all, I think it possibly depends on the kind of relationship you have'.

When required to justify their scepticism they point to the many marriages with children they know to have ended in divorce, and anyway, are they themselves not living proof of the proposition's falsity? They afford similarly scant consideration to the idea that children act as insurance against old age.

PARENTHOOD AS EMOTIONAL INSURANCE

Although the state may provide some form of financial insurance against hardship in old age, it does not provide any guarantee of emotional security: a hedge against loneliness, a source of companionship, of joy and support. The childless dismiss as selfish and callous the notion frequently expressed of bearing children to render this psychological service during old age.

Kate Tennant: 'A lot of our friends say, "Oh dear, what's going to happen if one of you goes and the other one's left? You're going to be so lonely. If only you had children"! I think that's a very selfish attitude.'

Kay Gregson: 'An awful lot of children give you an awful lot more heartache than enjoyment. I mean you just have to look about you, look at the country. You hear about an old woman dying in a house and not being found for three weeks . . . where's her children? A lot of people say they're good for your old age. I don't see how that's so. It's an awful hard way of looking at it – to just have children for when you're old.'

Kate Tennant and Kay Gregson found this lack of consideration for the child distasteful and echoed the words of Bob Adams who, rebelling against his mother's financial and psychological demands, refused to accept any other motive for having children than 'to give them pleasure and not want anything back in return'. If old age does mean loneliness, insecurity, and fear, then they will find the means for defence within themselves and will be prepared for the eventuality when it comes, a preparedness emerging out of awareness of the precarious nature of their exclusive relationships. Susan Dobie felt quite confident that 'by the time I'm left on my own, I'll adapt quite easily'.

Parenthood as emotional insurance is not specific to any social context; a similar meaning, parenthood as source of finance, is found only within a working-class or lower middle-class context. In the former it appears to be a case of 'what the child will contribute later'; in the latter a question of tax-relief. Motives that stress parental gain – whether material or psychological – are condemned as selfish and act to strengthen rather than weaken childless commitment by imbuing the latter with an aura of moral superiority quite at odds with the public image. Also deftly neutralized is the notion that parenthood proves sexual identity: that males are not masculine and females not feminine until they have performed in the reproductive arena.

PARENTHOOD AS PROOF OF SEXUAL IDENTITY

Jim McCausland: 'Look at the society at large, how does a man prove himself? First and most obvious is that he has kids. Well, that's changed slightly now, he drives a fast car, then he beats the piss out of everybody else around him in business . . . He's got a whole lot of ways of doing something about it. What the hell can a woman do? Have children and prove she's a woman, it's as simple as that.'

Married women without children run the risk of being labelled unfeminine: femininity implies maternity (Oakley 1982). Mary Johnson had first-hand experience of this equation: 'There's a woman in X . . . who insists you're not a woman until you've had a child'. Childless women tend strongly to object to this stereotype; the conventional image of the fertile as soft, compliant, yielding – femininity incarnate – and that of themselves as hard, brittle, and cold, are rejected as distorted and grossly oversimplified. Jeannie Maxwell: 'In fact some of the most feminine women I know even to-day are not married. They most probably have a most healthy sex-life but they don't have any children. It doesn't stop them being feminine'.

Childless women recognize that by neglecting to comply with one of the most salient features of the feminine image, they leave themselves open to the charge of having failed to realize their biological potential and therefore of being unfeminine. They nevertheless persist in their claim to femininity, basing it upon the assumption that being feminine is not solely a matter of participating in the reproductive process but is a complex of prescribed ways of acting, thinking, and feeling that together constitute womanhood. And it is upon their level of success in relation to these other aspects of the feminine image – particularly physical attractiveness – that they rest their claim. Success is measured in terms of masculine approval. More specifically, it is the husband whose support is crucial, according to Grace Simmons, 'As long as my husband thinks I'm feminine, that's all that matters'. Her husband's approval established and sustained the validity of her claim. In the words of Charles Quin, 'It's absolute, arrogant nonsense . . . it's impossible to say that because she hasn't got children she's not feminine . . . It's nonsense'.

Scant attention is similarly accorded cries of 'unnatural'; apart from the swift, almost contemptuous denial, refutation may take the form of a rhetorical question, 'What is natural?', and the *sequitur* that demands whether the unmarried and the celibate are also to be considered unnatural because of their failure to reproduce.

Such a failure on the part of the male leaves his sexual identity relatively unscathed. Not only is there no socially recognized paternal instinct with its accompanying claim to naturalness but the key – as Jim McCausland pointed out – to masculinity no longer lies in proof of virility through reproduction. The connection however may still be made and not exclusively by members of the working and lower middle classes where segregation of the sexes has been considered more marked. Ken Campbell, a TV engineer, suggested, 'Blokes show off – say it proves their virility'; whilst Bob McCormack, a self-employed professional, thought such behaviour rare, 'children of my own has never particularly appealed – as a demonstration of virility. I had one friend who had terrible hang-ups two years after he got married because he couldn't produce a child. He was the only one who considered it in that way – a slight upon his virility'.

As a motive for parenthood a desire to prove one's virility is dismissed as something of a joke, as a pathetic reminder of a chauvinist past in which women were used in the cause of masculine vanity. It assumes a way of perceiving self and relationship totally alien to the childless husband whose commitment to childlessness remains immune to this line of attack.

A similar lack of sympathy characterizes the childless response to the notion of parenthood as immortality.

PARENTHOOD AS IMMORTALITY

Children provide a link with the future; a hope of immortality. Creation implies joy and hope whilst the dream of immortality represents a profession of faith in tomorrow's world; when that faith ceases to exist, as it does for a number of childless men and women, creation may be perceived as an act of condemnation rather than the precious gift of life. Otherwise the childless – very much part of the here and now – tend to be barely conscious of parenthood's future orientation except to perhaps smile at the rarefied notion of carrying on the family name, a notion they come across in the media. For those who have no stake in the future it is the present that counts. There were couples however who, because of their material possessions, recognized why people like themselves might want to have children to 'follow on'.

Rory MacDonald: 'I must admit that I feel a twinge recently, I've said this to you several times . . . I'm always slightly depressed when you see something that someone had obviously cherished just simply being sold at an auction, you know. And I've said to Claire – I've got some vintage cars as well, and I've got a collection of books which is nice, which I've built up, we've got odds and ends of interesting, nice things and I've often said that it's a great pity that . . . there's no question they'll just have to be dispersed once we're dead and gone.'

The idea of parenthood as immortality may be fast becoming a 'relic of a superstitious past'; surviving in the bowdlerized notion of children as a material rather than psychic repository. One further victim to living for today appears to be the idea of parenthood as surrogate achievement.

PARENTHOOD AS SURROGATE ACHIEVEMENT

Parenthood may hold out the hope of an individual's achieving through his children what he himself will never achieve.

Sacrifices are made and ambitions killed to ensure a son's or even a daughter's greater success.

Christine Blake: 'The whole attitude of parenthood seems to be you get married and you have kids so you can bring your kids up to do all the things you would like to have done. And if you carry that to its natural conclusion no one's going to do anything after they're 35!'

The child is an investment, the returns being surrogate achievement, not financial gain. The childless reject this motive as another example of parental selfishness; the child is not wanted for its own sake but for the rewards it will bestow upon the parent caught up in the wake of a hoped-for success.

The childless label as immature, out-dated, and morally suspect the dominant motives informing reproductive behaviour. They insist that children should neither be the product of rational economic and psychic calculation nor the result of mindless conformity. All aspects of parenthood should however be given rational consideration and children conceived only if parents are convinced that their actions are informed by the purest of motives: to create and thereby give life to a human being who will be respected, loved, and cherished for himself. The childless – unless they themselves have looked forward eagerly to the prospect of parenthood – barely recognize notions of *parenthood as creation* and *as love* in the motives paraded before them. They do however concede that *parenthood as fun* and *children as bringers of joy* are meanings conveyed during the chivvying talk of the early stages of parenthood but that the realities of family life render these a less compelling argument for the parental role than the more self-centred motives paraded more openly. The childless therefore reject or neutralize dominant motives, an exercise that leaves their own reproductive commitment intact if not reinforced. They may be less successful when defending their position from direct attack. The cultural framework supports those who conform to reproductive expectations; it is the childless and not the parent whose actions are labelled selfish, immature, and wrong; consequently they develop various strategies to cope with this unsympathetic, at times hostile environment.

6

Childlessness:
the consequences of being different

Becoming and being a parent are experiences that people share. They are matters of common concern. The childless recognize that they cannot always escape enquiries about their parental status and that difficult questions may sometimes be asked. Their response depends upon the question, how it is asked, by whom and under what circumstances.

In informal encounters with comparative strangers, including old friends, they anticipate with varying degrees of resignation and resentment the inevitable query about whether or not they have children. Alan Dexter was quite philosophical, 'it's a more sophisticated version of when you meet an old friend, "It's hellish weather!" – it's a conversation-maker'. Interpreted in this way, the question is rarely resented; it is the response to a negative reply that is perceived as a likely source of tension. Questioners may demand further details that in the circumstances the childless may feel unable or unwilling to give. They believe their motives will not be accepted as valid; prevailing vocabularies of motive appear to define childlessness in purely negative terms. Each fresh encounter has to be managed carefully and with tact if both parties are to emerge unscathed.

Joan Ellison: 'People will say to you, "Do you have a family?" And I say, "No", and they sort of raise their eyebrows and I haven't said anything up until now . . . but I think I will soon. In fact I met somebody on Friday night and she was, you know, trying to get into it a bit and she got round and she was talking about her own family . . . I said I had no children and was about to launch off to see what her attitude would be but decided that it might launch into a sort of argument if I said I just don't want to have children or I don't see what difference it is going to make to my life to have children. She might get all het up about it and it might upset her. So I just thought, "Don't say anything".'

An alternative strategy frequently used with strangers is to divert their curiosity by admitting to having no children while at the same time inferring that attempts have been made or are about to be made to conceive (Veevers 1980). Even an un-equivocally negative response may be taken as an indication of sterility by individuals who adhere to the assumption that all normal married couples actively desire to become parents. The older the couple, the more likely the interpretation. Apart from half-hearted jibes at the male's sexual prowess, it is women who take the brunt of these insinuations demonstrated in the swift, embarrassed change of subject, the gesture of pity – 'in a look' – and most intrusive of all, the request for physical details and full medical history.

Brenda Oliver: 'I met this woman on a bus and I got talking to her. I know her very vaguely but not particularly – she's not even a friend of my mother as such but I know her to speak to – I've known her for a long time in that sense. This was only about two years after we were married, she said to me, "Oh, have you any family yet?" I said, "No". She said, "Oh, what's the matter with you?" I don't think I had an answer to that, I was dumbfounded.'

As Brenda Oliver's reaction suggests, irritation and anger at this invasion of privacy is compounded by the difficulty individuals have in retaliating given context and questioner. In contrast the more commonplace query as to parental status is tolerated; it is a legitimate question in an encounter where sociability is the aim and individuals interact more or less as equals. Even an innocuous enquiry may appear threatening where an individual feels under pressure to conform and may cause distress by heightening existing feelings of isolation and guilt: an infrequent reaction experienced by women and only during the early stages of commitment.

When sterility is not assumed, a negative response may elicit demands as to intentions. This information may be offered freely and truthfully in an act of defiance. Ian Donaldson: 'Some people assume you do have them and are quite surprised when you say you haven't. They're even more surprised when you say you've no intention having any which I sometimes say just to shock them'. Such a direct assault upon basic beliefs may be met by further demands for explanation. The childless feel they cannot explain and will attempt to avoid not only committing themselves but also committing others to this awkward situation. Alan Dexter: 'One doesn't discuss it to be perfectly honest because you never know unless the other person says first, you never know you aren't going to offend them mortally by attacking their virility or social awareness'. Evasion may prove unnecessary since a comparative stranger may recoil from the implications of further questioning. Even when they volunteer their intentions, the childless may go unchallenged; they are simply not believed. Diane Marshall was not alone in finding this reaction patronizing:

'Now I just don't bother saying anything unless they say something because I have had some arguments with people . . . they very condescendingly say, "Oh, when I was young I thought that. I've got three lovely boys now". That's the most common – a patronizing attitude, "Oh, you'll change your mind when you get older. I thought that but now I've got my children I wouldn't do without them and I don't know how I existed before"!'

These comments form part of the recruitment drive. Glaser and Strauss (1971) have described how the recruiter may idealize a status passage for the potential recruit who appears reluctant to embark upon it. The reassuring utterances directed at the childless during their most eligible years appear to serve this function. It is taken for granted that their eventual conformity is simply a matter of time, a question of growing up. Chivvying is intended to hasten this process. Explanation is not required; immaturity is the obvious answer.

Questioning may persist but be met by indignation and lack of cooperation from the childless, who feel cornered by an inability to call upon a set of accepted motives and perceiving the encounter as yet another invasion of privacy, swiftly bring it to a close; on the other hand, they may wish to make their case but to avoid conflict carefully match motives to audience and situation. The least inflammatory meanings are proffered: a dislike for children, an altruistic wish not to add to the world's population problem.

Diane Marshall: 'Last year on holiday I was talking to this chap and he was saying how long have you been married and all this – and you've no children . . . "When are you intending to have one?" . . . eventually I got fed up and said, "We're not intending to have any" . . . Oh, you should have seen him, you know, "Oh, you'll grow out of that, you'll change your attitude". When I finally got across the point that I wouldn't change my attitude and it wasn't just a phase I was going through he said, "Oh, do your parents know?" And I said, "No". And he said, "They'll be terribly disappointed". I said, "You don't have children just to suit other people". And I said, "Well anyway who'd want to bring children into this world". No, he was so optimistic, man's been in this position before and all the rest of it, there's always been the prophets of doom. I said, "We've never been in a position as bad as this before". "Oh", he said, "give me an example". I said, "Well, for instance, energy". And he said, "But my firm's experimenting with a new type of battery". I thought, "Oh, my God!" He thought it was the answer to the world's energy problems.'

Diane Marshall would be the first to admit that the state of the world and the population problem are for her a convenient justification. They can and do prove to be motives that others accept as legitimate even though they may not share the same convictions. This basis for understanding may be used to ease tension and may even make childlessness a more viable alternative. In intellectual circles, it appears rather fashionable to forego parenthood for humanity's sake. According to Tom

Irvine, a university lecturer, 'Of course working in a university everyone is swinging in on environmental problems and it becomes a virtue to be childless'. Nevertheless motives that others are perceived incapable of accepting, that infringe too blatantly beliefs that sanctify the family, that are considered too intimate for public exposure, remain for the most part locked within the marital realtionship occasionally to be disclosed to a select few. Casual encounters do not call for such unmasking.

Martin Todd: 'We used to put much more emphasis on the dreadful future that one would be bringing children into . . . I don't think we'd ever have said that we felt it was somehow an imposition on our privacy and solitude or way of life . . . I used to say to people I hated kids . . .'

During these encounters individuals expect and receive little sympathy and support. Faced with an image of themselves as selfish, immature, unnatural, weird, odd, they may attempt to mask their identity, to evade awkward questions, to manage situations which for some women at least are a trial, if not an ordeal. Others may attack but none retreat. Reactions monitored in fleeting, casual encounters may not dent childless commitment and may actively reinforce it whilst at the same time confirming what the childless perceive as unwarranted prejudice.

Martin Todd: 'The worst thing about not having children is being considered some kind of weird freak by the vast majority of the population.'
Patricia Campbell: 'Many people . . . a neighbour next door thinks I'm weird – I overheard a conversation and there was a girl at work who asked, "Is she alright?" – because I didn't have a baby.'

The childless reject these images that are a constant reminder of their difference. One means they have of counter-attack is to discredit the critic (Veevers 1980); members of the recruitment drive are seen as trying to foist on to others tasks they have found onerous and unrewarding. Douglas Johnson: 'It's generally people who've – I think there's a bit of sadism involved here – because it's people who've had kids and haven't had a good time

with them that want to inflict them on other people'. When not
sadists, they may be dismissed as the unthinking mass. Critical
opinion is therefore registered but painlessly neutralized with
minimal damage; hostility on the part of friends and relatives
may be less easily parried. A parent's desire for grandchildren
might be considered one of the major stumbling-blocks to a
couple's choosing the childless way of life.

Henry Blair: 'The only people I would say one was being selfish to
in not having children were parents who wanted to become
grandparents. Now in our case both lots of parents have
become grandparents . . . So I'm not worried about that.'

The childless do not doubt the attraction grandchildren hold for
their parents – only two mothers appeared hostile to the prospect
– but little pressure was openly exerted. Questions may be asked,
particularly once the postponement period has extended beyond
its normal limits, at which point parents, perhaps anxious and
impatient, may attempt to chivvy their children into action.

Mary Fraser: 'I suppose they must have . . . they did, they . . . not
so much my own mother, but Colin's mother did, she said
several times, "Nothing happening, no news?" . . . But to be
perfectly fair to her she has never nagged about it or said
anything for a long time . . . certainly several times in the
earlier years of our marriage she did ask but that was all. She
did once say, "Have you seen about it?" '

These efforts may be forestalled by couples dropping hints that
leave parents in no doubt as to their intentions but even when
left in the dark parents do not automatically bombard their
children with a barrage of questions and criticisms. This
restraint may in fact be an accurate reading of the response they
would get if they were to probe.

Charles Quin: 'I don't consider it is anybody's business, including
parents . . . my parents certainly haven't mentioned it, they
haven't said, "Come on, where's the grandchild?", sort of
thing. And I would tell them it wasn't any of their business if
they did because I don't consider it is.'

Charles Quin was not close to his parents. Others were, and tried to avoid conflict by simply not raising the question of their childlessness. Parents, they believed, recognized their position and kept a diplomatic silence. Parenthood becomes taboo – allowing those involved to defuse situations potentially harmful to their relationship. The recognition of a need to tread warily may result in parents masking their interest and concern behind a façade of joking and teasing (Goffman 1961).

Claire MacDonald: 'I'm really very close to my parents . . . And I know they would like a grandchild. Mummy, she'd never say it to me and make me feel terrible. In fact she's never said it but I know she would. And father used to say, "I wouldn't mind being a grandfather" – jokingly.'

When they neither joke nor tease – unsure of their ground perhaps but wanting to express their feelings – parents restrict themselves to mild comment; rarely do couples feel under pressure. Ellen Kennedy's description of her father as 'always on at me about not having a family' is unusual. A number of couples believed they had escaped a concerted attack by living at a distance from their parents. Distance appears to transform what would be pressure into at worst a minor aggravation that may be treated as a joke.

Philip Tennant: 'Your mother at one stage she went on at us till we were blue in the face about it, dropping hints and gentle reminders.'
Kate Tennant: ' "What are you doing about it?" . . . And "Remember that friend that you used to know she's just had her third baby". "Oh, has she mother?" If I was on the phone to my mother and I'd say, "I'm not feeling very well, hang-over from the week-end". She had me pregnant. Absolutely thrilled at the thought of it. "Have you been to the doctor, dear?" "No, you don't go to the doctor if you have a hang-over, Mum" . . . I wouldn't say it was a problem. Okay, it got annoying.'
Philip Tennant: 'I think it would have been very hard to withstand the pressures if your mother had been living on the doorstep.'

Geographical distance not only dilutes pressures but renders parrying tactics more effective; these attempts to avoid disclosure may be made not simply to protect the childless themselves but to shield the parent who might be shocked and hurt by an admission of voluntary childlessness.

If it is the childless who are vulnerable, parrying is replaced by an obvious annoyance or hostile silence intended to convey an unwillingness to talk and to issue a warning that the topic is taboo. Jacqueline Webster: 'My mother has said that Andrew's mother was on about it. I've said, "Oh, was she?" and the conversation ends there from the look on my face. I don't want to discuss it with my mother'. When disclosures are made, immediate reactions – although varying considerably between indifference, disbelief, disappointment and support – are generally restrained. Disbelief is the least common response and is found only amongst the parents of couples only recently married or who share some mitigating circumstance such as an unhappy pregnancy history. Otherwise they appear to respect the sincerity of the childless intention; disappointed, some make it quite clear they neither understand nor approve of the decision.

Martin Todd: 'Mother always has a little niggle, doesn't she?'
Lesley Todd: 'She's not a silly woman in some ways but she's very emotional and she's very affectionate and the fact that her first son is married and got a wife that she likes and things. We're both healthy and intelligent and all the rest of it and she thinks it's sad that we don't want children.'

As the many references to mothers suggest, having children is predominantly a feminine concern, consequently, it is mainly mothers who feel cheated, affronted by the unconventional behaviour of their children and unable to compete on equal terms with other women. This reaction is particularly acute amongst women who do not already have grandchildren and whose only hope lies with the childless couple. Martin Todd explains his situation, 'My sister . . . she's been trying to have children and hasn't managed it and . . . as a result I think my mother has been rather heavy on us sometimes . . .' Other parents may be able to curb their disappointment and offer support and encouragement. A few applaud the decision and even defend and espouse their children's cause. But, as in Carol

Blair's case, support is tinged more often than not by a rarely expressed sadness, 'My mother, I think, would have liked us to have them but never really thought that we would . . . I think she thinks we have satisfying careers and in our case it would be a mistake'.

When the decision has registered, its rationale is rarely questioned; parents tend not to demand explanations – if they wonder, they do so in private. If asked for an opinion, they express their reservations whilst making it quite clear it is not *their* life nor *their* commitment. Meaningful dialogue appears most likely to occur between mothers and daughters where both have doubts not only about motherhood but about the feminine role in general. Carol Thompson had gained considerable support from her mother who shared her desire for freedom and self-determination:

> 'She particularly thinks it's good . . . she always says if she had a life to live again she wouldn't be married . . . one night we were sitting here and I said, "If I'm coming back I'm coming back a man. They've got a great life". My mother said, "If I had my time to live again, I wouldn't be married" . . . This is what she'd want and she said, "You have one life, live it as you want to. If you feel you've got married and you don't want children, don't have children. But get as much happiness out of your life as you can".'

But where mother and daughter hold conflicting views, disaffection from the feminine role – even when a salient consideration – is not always proffered or so readily accepted as a motive for rejecting motherhood. Targets for and elements of confessions are carefully chosen since childless women in particular are well aware of the labels – abnormal, odd, unnatural – that are frequently and indiscriminately attached to those who step outside what is conventionally prescribed. But whereas the 'public at large' may be generally quick to abuse and accuse, parents, no less cognizant of the negative imagery surrounding childlessness, tread more warily and moderate the expression of any doubts they may entertain as to the wisdom of the childless intent and the normality of their children. It would appear to be the absence of any positive image or set of acceptable motives that silences demands for and offers of explanation. Both sides seem to recognize that any attempt to go beyond the simple statement of intent might result in spiralling misunderstanding and possible breakdown of the relationship. Relationships, however, can and do survive these episodes of enlightenment: an outcome which to a certain extent reflects the level of censorship applied. Motives are selected for communication according to the degree of understanding and acceptance likely to be involved. Couples tend to stress the distasteful and sacrificial aspects of parenthood and the relative freedoms of remaining childless. Both positions are liable to rejection; but both can be understood. Wanting to please oneself may be defined as 'selfish' and morally reprehensible within a cultural framework that projects an image of parenthood as duty and that demands parental sacrifice. Yet at the same time it is understandable since this same framework enjoins and applauds the acquisition of material, physical, and psychic pleasures and stresses the individual's right to pursue his own destiny. The sin the childless commit is to abuse this right by choosing a destiny that by-passes what appears to be a higher value: parenthood. Also the norm of parental sacrifice is so deeply embedded in the adult consciousness that even the childless appear uncertain as to whether their actions justify the 'selfish' label. It is little wonder, therefore, that some parents see their children as 'cold', 'calculating' and 'callous'. Disapproval of this motive, however is not universal; here and there parents congratulate their children on a wise and sensible decision. But most parents, having survived the rigours of child-care, stand by the public image.

They may be willing to admit that it 'wasn't all plain-sailing' while claiming it was 'well worth it'. A case based upon distaste receives little sympathy: a dirty nappy phobia, however real, makes a feeble excuse for abrogating so important a responsibility. The reaction, although understandable given the unpleasant nature of some aspects of child-care – a point generally conceded by parents – is countered by the attitude, 'If we could do it, so can you'. An excess of sensitivity, when persisted in, is likely to be interpreted as a sign of immaturity or some other weakness of character that brings out the smile which seems to say, 'when you grow up . . .' Able and willing to accept such a response, the childless may use distaste for the tasks of child-care or dislike for children to ward off the curious parent. They may remain, however, unwilling to expose more important motives they believe parents incapable of understanding; the reason for this interpretive fissure they perceive as lying with parental adherence to a perspective that has marriage, parenthood, and the family as an indivisible, inviolable trinity. The childless by definition reject this 'limited' vision; parents mean well, they are simply misguided in their acceptance of a public image their children have the foresight to see beyond; the views they express can therefore be discounted as those of a past generation now out of touch.

Although most parents show some interest in the reproductive activities of their children and experience varying degrees of disappointment when the outcome appears to be no grand-children, they have nearly all reached a stage in the family life-cycle where parenthood is no longer a central concern. Changing interests reflect in conversation; when children are no longer an immediate responsibility talk is less likely to focus upon the multi-faceted parental role. It is the expectant and new parent who, according to the childless, tends to dwell upon the joys and delights of parenthood.

Graham Marshall: 'And even the blokes . . . especially young blokes who've recently had children. "You don't know what you're missing" . . . "Oh, it's great to have a lad to play with".'
Ellen Vernon: 'They go on and on about it . . . "Oh, I do hope Mike makes a lot of money then you can leave work and have children and stay at home like the rest of us".'

The recruitment drive gathers strength as more couples join the parental ranks and those without children become the odd ones out. It is generally assumed that conformity is only a matter of time. Talk is therefore a form of incentive to action. This not too subtle attempt at persuasion is recognized by the childless, ever-sensitive to anything that might be construed as a critical cue. Susan Dobie had little time for her friend's insinuations: 'And sometimes it irritates me because she goes on about her own family so much that I don't know whether this is a sort of hint but I take it to be a hint and I get peeved sometimes'.

On the other hand parents who may be simply trying to come

to terms with a new, exciting, and often puzzling obsession may inadvertently succeed in talking any childless friend into a state of petrified boredom from which the relationship may never recover. Although most friendships appear to survive this period of child over-kill, they may do so only to succumb under the weight of curiosity that manifests itself in a constant stream of questions directed at those couples whose postponement has violated the strictures of the reproductive timetable. Amongst friends the discussion of parenthood appears to be something of a ritualistic free flow of information: a reflection of the 'we're all in this together' attitude that informs the chivvying tactics of earlier rounds. Reproductive histories and experiences, duly whitewashed, are pooled as public property. Images circulate and myths are perpetuated. Meanwhile, the childless are expected to participate in these consolidatory activities by responding to the friendly promptings of the curious and concerned. Only those with a family history of sterility – biographical information often available to friends – or who marry so late as to be ineligible, escape enquiry and avoid the decision of whether or not to reveal their commitment. No more than ties of kinship does friendship guarantee understanding, forbearance, and a swift, uncompromising denial of the dominant imagery. One strategy is to say nothing and to allow others to interpret the silence. Such an approach appears to demand on the one hand, patience from the childless, and on the other, only muted curiosity on the part of friends. Where these conditions hold, by simply sitting out the storm, couples find that questions die a natural death with familiarity and the passage of time. Couples become accepted and identified as childless. Joan Ellison had had to wait six years for 'people to get used to the fact that we haven't any children'.

Similarly accepted are couples where one or both partners had made a well-publicized and insistent pre-marital commitment.

Questions become something of a formality: a joking reminder of a quirk in an otherwise sound character.

Liz Finlay: 'People just accept the fact, probably 'cos they've known I've never wanted children for years . . . I mean I think most people have known my attitude through the years. Whenever children have been mentioned I've gone,

"Ugh!" . . . People keep saying "Have you not changed your mind yet?" And I keep saying, "No" . . . They're joking with you rather than pressing you.'

On the other hand, couples who appear normal are considered legitimate targets for comment when desultory in their reproductive efforts. Attempts to stall and feign sterililty – appropriate in the fleeting relationship – may prove impossible to handle where the context is friendship.

Kate Tennant: 'I took the coward's way out because I announced to all my friends I could not have children.'
Philip Tennant: ' "Isn't it a pity . . ." '
Kate Tennant: ' ". . . we can't have children", which of course killed . . . they stopped asking. And then after a time it was pretty obvious I was on the pill, swallowing it like mad. I had to tell the truth after a while.'
Philip Tennant: 'I've heard you tell both stories on the same evening to the same person.'
Kate Tennant: 'But it was a coward's way out 'cos I got so fed up with people saying, "Why don't you have children, we all do?".'

The breathing space gained at the expense of hushed tones and pitying glances helps protect an embryonic commitment that might otherwise give under the weight of friendly persuasion. In only one case did these efforts have any direct impact upon behaviour.

Marjorie Nelson: 'I think only once – Stella got through to me in X 'cos she was out there at the same time as us and she used to keep on – it was day-in, day-out, day-in, day-out she'd keep on about having a kid. Once I said to him, "Come on, let's try", but that lasted all of two hours!'
Robert Nelson: 'Let's be honest, you said you'd give it a try for a month. Looking back on it, it was bloody ridiculous. She'd been on the pill for three-and-a-half to four years, she stopped it for one month, then she'd go back on the pill – built-in immunization and the fact that she didn't want one anyway.'
Marjorie Nelson: 'I really didn't give it any thought. I said to him –

I'd got so fed up with Stella that I said, "Okay, Stella, I'll give it a try for a month". That shut her up and I came off the pill for a month but it never entered my head that I'd have no more chance than a snow-ball in hell . . . I think I'd have probably killed myself if I'd found I was pregnant. That was beside the point but at best it shut her up.'

This is an extreme but highly effective strategy for silencing critics but one most couples feel loath to take. Friends may be annoying, but not a problem. If relations become over-strained, the friendship may be allowed to cool and eventually peter out: a victim to diverging interests and therefore no loss. Less easy for the childless to accept is the failure of friends to whom they do confide to accept the legitimacy of their position. Disbelief and misunderstanding are common responses but so also is the reinterpretation of the childless intent – in spite of all protestations to the contrary – as a couple's attempt to hide the 'real' and 'unhappy' reason for their failure to conform – sterility.

Carol Blair: 'With some other (friends) I would say they couldn't really understand why I didn't want children, they thought I was compensating by going to the university, you know, doing something new and that sort of thing . . . And also we had a dog at the time – I baby substituted!'

Everything this childless couple do is seen as confirming the validity of the sterile definition; hence the dog becomes a living proof of the couple's failed attempts at parenthood. The image imposed is of husband and wife striving to fill an empty existence with constant and vacuous activity. Even where a couple are accorded credibility, the rationality they impute to their action may be rejected in favour of an interpretation that maintains the integrity of the Siamese-twin-like relationship between the marital and parental roles by explaining their behaviour as a weakness of character on the part of one or other or both partners. Odd, unnatural, weird, unfeminine/ unmasculine, are labels the bonds of friendship do not automatically neutralize – they rather generate a sifting process whereby characteristics are selected that fit the childless friend(s) in question. Jeannie Maxwell: 'I get on terribly well with men. And of course I've been told by two of my friends the reason I do this is I'm trying to prove I really am feminine because I don't have any children'. The woman is most frequently considered abnormal, rejecting, as she does, an identity that dominates the lives of her contemporaries. The emphasis, however, quickly changes and childlessness for both men and women may come to represent a sad omission that friends politely ignore, quietly pity and from time to time challenge in the hope of conversion. Kate Tennant: 'People said very quickly, "Phil and Kate aren't going to have kids, aren't they missing a lot, poor souls?" And they felt sorry for us'.

Couples with children, but more particularly women who adhere more or less to traditional expectations, may assume an air of superiority towards their childless friends. If a woman is not a woman until she becomes a mother, in the eyes of the latter the childless woman has not proven her right to equal feminine status.

Edwina McCausland: 'Women who were not as intelligent as I could overnight after having a baby immediately adopt a totally superior attitude because they had had a baby and if I hadn't had a baby then I knew nothing about nothing.'

These women draw their superiority from an image of femininity reinforced by an army of supportive prescriptions and values. Their disdain, together with the disbelief and pity others express, reflect the normality of parenthood. Childlessness is a form of aberration. This notion absolves them – incriminated by association – and their rather odd friends from blame. The childless, deemed not responsible for their unhappy situation, as victims do not pose a threat to the family image and are therefore to be pitied rather than censured. If they were to be accorded rational choice, this concession would bring into question the naturalness and inevitability of parenthood. The filtering through of rationality into the instinctive reaches of reproduction may engender uncertainty and insecurity in those, and more obviously women, it touches. Its prophets – amongst them the voluntarily childless – may therefore be greeted defensively by those no longer assured of the natural image. This uncertainty may presage the metamorphosis of the unitary family image into a kaleidoscopic array of alternative forms; less dramatically, it may also reflect a mere transition to a modified but still triumphant unit of husband, wife, children where meanings and motives may have changed but where the foundation itself remains unmoved. Parents who are aware of, even if they have not experienced the effects of these disturbing trends upon their own lives, may empathize with those couples who opt out by remaining childless.

Carol Blair: 'They (husband's colleagues and friends) do understand that people can genuinely think like that. John, for example, he has children and he just accepts it. He doesn't think one way or the other.'

This understanding seemingly restricted to the unconventional middle class may be supplemented by the support of friends who are childless. Where childless friends meet childless friends mutuality of interest is recognized and discussion consolidatory. Friendships such as these are not easily made. The childless couple tend to see themselves as socially isolated. Husband and wife together form a barren island amidst a sea of reproductive activity. It is not that they are without friendship; what they may lack and what generates this feeling of isolation is any real understanding from friends on the specific question of their childlessness. Childlessness becomes increasingly private; being turned inward upon themselves underlines their differentness and may prompt the question: 'Have you ever come across anybody like us?'. Even the friendship of other childless couples fails to assuage this awareness of being different and of being considered by all and sundry, including many friends, at best, misguided.

Cathy McCormack: 'I think they are probably in a way right. Not right in my mode of thinking but right in the way they've been brought up. If you think of the way we've all been brought up, to feel as I feel is abnormal. It's not, it wasn't accepted . . . I think in the next twenty years if things like you're doing work, people will think it's not abnormal. But at the moment people who say this are right in their own way. In our terms of thinking, in our environment it is abnormal to get married and not have children. But thinking is coming round to the fact that it is not abnormal.'

Labels may be perceived as legitimate but not accepted. The most frequent reaction to friends who choose to cast doubt upon their normality is to assert the contrary; this belief in themselves and the legitimacy of their commitment, is sustained by a number of counter-interpretations.

Where the childless perceive their commitment as attributable to favourable circumstances, labels are understood as the uninformed response of the less fortunate, and are discounted and defied. This is a stand taken by the professional middle class who may reinterpret their differentness as being in the vanguard and not as abnormality. Their reaction to friends who have yet to recognize childlessness as part of the future is one of understanding; they make no effort to correct the false interpretation of their motives, they appear to sit back as if waiting to be vindicated by a revolution in reproductive norms. Neither of these reactions – stemming from a deep-seated belief in the legitimacy of a childless way of life – is common even amongst members of the professional middle class.

The most frequent reaction to the conventional outpourings of friends is a tight-lipped good humour generally confined to the privacy of the marital relationship where husband and wife together wage what is for them a functional counter-attack. Pity, although generally recognized as a simple parody of conventional wisdom, they see as merely misplaced when not obviously a veiled condemnation. They look at themselves and at these pitying friends, a comparison which acts to heighten their awareness of the factors that have destined others for parenthood whilst they remain childless. Christine Blake: 'There are a lot of people that are really happy about having children but they're not the same people as us by any means, they're people that have settled down'. Pity they explain as arising from their friends' inability to see that a life without children may have its own satisfactions and that these may be the object of rational choice. Pity is a response born of convention and not of rational consideration; it can therefore be discounted as one link in the process of perpetuating family myth. Outflanked by the power of the latter's tenacious imagery, the childless tend to shun what

they see as the thankless task of accounting for their commitment. Amongst those few who make the effort are a small
number of crusading spirits intent on increasing awareness
whilst also liberalizing the childless image (These same goals
were espoused by the National Association for the Childless and
Childfree, formed in England in the mid-70s but whose existence
had not yet filtered through to these Scottish couples.) Their goal
is reproductive freedom of choice; to achieve it they reveal all
aspects of their commitment. They see openness as the key to
wider acceptance of the childless alternative and to the destruc-
tion of the cultural fastness that protects the nuclear family. So
candid an approach is restricted to those with a mission; less
candid are those who cash in on existing imagery by using the
stereotypes as a form of defiance intended to thwart the carping
of those who lace their pity and disdain with implied if not stated
accusations of selfishness. Kate Tennant: 'I used to say I work.
That shocked everybody!' Even where pity is qualified the
childless are still perceived as victims but victims who are
over-compensated for their failings by an excess of freedom,
pleasure, money, and 'things'. Being deviant is seen to pay – and
to pay handsomely. The childless interpret these accusations as
'sour grapes', indicative of the envy their friends with children
cannot help but experience when they recognize the advantages
of remaining childless.

Susan Dobie: 'We use this couple for comparison. Talking about
   holidays, just looking at them, they can't go for holidays, they
   haven't been on a holiday for years. They just can't get up and
   go when they want. I think sometimes they're very jealous of
   us because we've got this ability to get up and go when we
   want.'
Sandra O'Neill: 'I think a lot of my friends are slightly jealous
   because they know I can up and away and help Jim or whatever's going on at the time.'

From the vantage point of their chosen way of life the childless
couple greet such demonstrations of jealousy not with resentment but with a tolerant and knowing smile. Envy they perceive
as a begrudging recognition of the wisdom of their choice. In
time however the jealousy abates, the indignation and disdain

burns out, the pity subsides, and the couple become just that – a couple.

Sandra O'Neill: 'They don't (ask) now. Most of my friends they've had their one and I joke, "I think I'm pregnant". "What you, I can't imagine you pregnant!" . . . they'd find it odd if I suddenly started pushing a pram up the street . . . they just accept us as Sandra and Jimmy O'Neill.'

They survive the onslaught – commitment intact and frequently enhanced by an attachment born of growing awareness – to find that they have created a self-sufficient unit impervious to the judgement of an unsympathetic world.

7

Maintaining commitment:
strategies of control

Having committed themselves to childlessness and remaining sexually active, couples face the practical difficulties of controlling their fertility. The methods from which they can choose include the various contraceptive techniques, sterilization, and abortion. The strategies they opt for depend to a large extent upon the constraints of individual commitment, i.e. whether it is provisional or total, and is based on rejection of parenthood or attachment to childlessness. But whatever the qualifications and amendments to basic commitment, while continuing to define themselves as voluntarily childless, all couples aim to prevent conception. The levels of effectiveness of the more modern forms of contraception virtually eliminate accidental pregnancy that is not attributable to human error. The contraceptive pill is at the centre of this reproductive revolution and it is in the pill's apparent infallibility that a majority of the childless place their trust. The promise of security it offers may even wear down the 'prejudices and misapprehensions' of women who began married life before it was generally available, but who, as time passes, become more fearful of the effects of motherhood upon a way of life to which they have become increasingly attached. Carol Blair, in her late 30s with a job she enjoys and a satisfactory marriage, had found herself in this situation:

'I think I should be on the pill because the nerves . . . it's just not really worth the worry sometimes . . . Henry doesn't believe in the pill . . . we used to use the cap, but we haven't used that for a while. We generally use the sheath now . . . it's certainly not a satisfactory solution.'

For Carol Blair as well as for members of the pill generation, the pill's acceptability rests first and foremost in its reliability. Other factors that have been found to affect a method's acceptability such as availability, cost, safety, aesthetics (Bone 1973) pale in significance besides this one overriding criterion. Even when experienced, side-effects that have become part of the culture of pill-taking tend to be given scant consideration and dismissed as normal, 'nothing to worry about', or as a minor irritation. Rosemary Hall: 'I've never had any side-effects except I've put on about a stone in weight but I think everybody does. Over seven years it's not bad really'. The pill becomes a fact of life written into the daily routine. Rosemary Hall again: 'I would stay on the pill forever. It's a habit. It's like brushing your teeth. To me it is, brush my teeth and take my pill at the same time'. Side-effects cannot always be so easily shrugged off, but even severe migraine, persistent headaches, and other discomforts may still be an acceptable price to pay for peace of mind. The benefits of reliability outweigh the costs to general health.

Brenda Oliver: 'This pill's all right and it's a lot better than the previous brand – I've been lucky, they've been really helpful up at the FPA, super – because I'm one of those people that everything upsets – I retain fluid, the lot. So they've juggled me around from pill to pill, but this one I'm on now isn't bad.'
Allan Oliver: 'It does have side-effects but there could be a worse side-effect and nothing else has the same sureness.'

Only when reliability is bought at too high a price will women turn to what they see as less attractive methods such as the diaphragm and sheath. Not only is the pill reliable, it is also more pleasant to use.

Christine Blake: 'It'd be okay if I could take the pill. I tried that . . . oh, for about a year, it was terrible. I was getting migraines. It was at the stage I was taking three days off in a month because I just couldn't get out of bed . . . And I put on about a stone in a

month. It just wasn't worth it because what's the point if you
just don't feel like doing it. I felt like a monster. The cap's a bit
sort of cumbersome. We're adjusted to it but we still feel it's a
bit of a nuisance.'

Young women compelled to make this substitution saw it as an
interim arrangement; the loss of reliability and spontaneity
being unacceptable in anything but the short term. (The cap
did have its champion: a 39-year-old woman who had used it
effectively for 10 years and who described herself as 'too set in
my ways' to change to the pill, that was anyway 'not for me'.)
Similarly, where the highly effective loop takes the place of the
pill, though without the unpleasant aspects of the sheath and cap,
it has the disadvantages of painful insertion and the possibility
of regular replacement and check-ups, which for women using it
were obvious drawbacks, rendering it a stop-gap measure.

Patricia Campbell: 'I was thinking next year I'll go back to the
   Clinic . . . and ask about sterilization. I think you have to get it
   (loop) changed every year and in that case – I didn't enjoy it
   going in, it was quite painful – I might get sterilized. They can
   take this loop out while I'm under anaesthetic, thank you very
   much! . . . there's no point if I don't want a baby to go every
   year and get this loop changed because it is quite painful for
   someone who hasn't had a baby to have it put in. Discomfort
   lasted about – the first three days were agony and it lasted
   about a week – pain.'

If commitment is total, sterilization is the obvious alternative;
the problem then becomes one of availability. If, on the other
hand, it remains provisional, sterilization becomes an option
only if the fear of conception heightened by having to use a new
and supposedly inadequate method is not minimized by the
back-up strategy of abortion: abortion is recognized as available
but unacceptable. The Blakes, a couple in their early 20s finding
themselves in this situation, believed they had little choice but to
redefine their commitment as total and seek sterilization.

Christine Blake: 'I don't suppose if I'd been on the pill we'd have
   come to this decision.'

John Blake: 'We want to make it final because we don't want to go on without sterilization of some kind until we're thirty-five or something because the most important time for us not to have kids is now. If an accident happened now we'd be bombed out completely.'

Similarly not all women taking the pill are happy with their situation and carefree in the knowledge of the method's apparent infallibility. Initially Sheila Kidd worried incessantly, and now, 'I still can't accept the pill as a complete protection – I don't care what any medical person says. I'm not as bad now as I was, I don't check it every minute'. Jacqueline Webster was annoyed that 'you have to remember to take the pill every night . . . My memory is getting worse. You've got to remember. If you're sick and you bring it up, that's that. A girl-friend of mine fell pregnant through a tummy upset. You have to re-member all these little things to make it 100 per cent safe'. Nor do women always experience side-effects with stoicism and equanimity. Kay Gregson: 'I worry a lot about what I'll look like when I'm 40. Like the pill, I've put on about one-and-a-half stones, it really depresses me'. These women perceive the pill as less than infallible, and its side-effects problematic because they have already recognized in sterilization an acceptable and reliable alternative; gone would be the one thousand to one chance of accidental pregnancy, anxiety over memory-lapse, unpleasant side-effects, and fears of long-term usage, but gone also would be the opportunity to conceive, of reversing com-mitment to childlessness. Acceptance of sterilization there-fore depends upon total commitment.

Betty Hamilton: 'I would be quite prepared to undergo sterilization although the doctor explained that they wouldn't consider you until you are in your late 20s – they don't feel you can make that kind of decision until you are that age – I feel at the moment I could. I can't see any reason to make me change my mind in the future and I would be quite happy to be sterilized . . . I think as I get older my attitude will become more and more definite. People don't seem to realize that once you have made up your mind to do something, then that's it. I feel I am making the right decision.'

Not everyone shares this level of certainty. Rosemary Hall, now 30, recognizes the possibility of reversing her commitment – however remote:

> 'At my age and the way things are just now I have no intentions of having any children. But at the same time I would never be sterilized – the medical side of it, that's nothing to do with it, but I always think to myself, "You never know, maybe you'll change, something might make you change". I think it's too final. Certainly I wouldn't be sterilized myself nor would I expect my husband to be sterilized because I think the age of the father is less important than the age of the mother . . . I could be killed to-morrow, he could get married to somebody else and really want to have children . . . So I think it's too final.'

While any doubt remains, individuals like Rosemary Hall are unwilling to foreclose their options; uncertainty however recedes with age. Women in particular tend to relate the acceptability of sterilization to loss of reproductive eligibility and set an age-limit between the early to late 30s after which they will be unsuitable for motherhood and sterilization the most convenient form of control. Liz Finlay, for example, 'wouldn't take the chance of having any' after 34; not only did she believe she would be unable to meet the demands of a small infant but also that the older she was, the greater the likelihood of that infant being in some way deformed. Both ideas appear central to notions of eligibility. Age-limits were also set by women and some husbands who feared the effects of long-term pill usage but even these fears were insufficient to deter women from maintaining voluntary commitment. Ellen Vernon, a research biologist, was particularly philosophical about her situation:

> 'It doesn't really worry me being on the pill for most of my life. Okay, so it may increase your risk of dying in one particular way by a certain amount but, you know, you've got to die of something and you may die crossing the road to-morrow, so . . . I'd rather go on taking the pill until the menopause than have you sterilized – in case I change my mind.'

Where freedom of choice outweighs both long and short-term costs, sterilization is unacceptable; the problem arises where one partner continues to express reservations whilst the other is totally committed and favours sterilization.

Allan Oliver: 'Brenda feels she may change her mind . . . Quite honestly I'd go and get sterilized to-morrow if it wasn't – quite honestly you feel you may change your mind later on. I don't feel I ever will, I feel fairly convinced in myself although need-less to say, I can't be 100 per cent.'

Brenda Oliver: 'I'm keeping it open . . . I know I've changed a lot since I was 16 to now, so I could change a lot from now till I'm 30 but the truth is, it's not a very satisfactory way to go on. Allan said he would think about sterilization but for me and it's a problem because you've really got to think. I don't want to turn round in five years' time and say, "Oh, you shouldn't have done that. You should have left it".'

Allan Oliver had conceded to his wife's uncertainty. Parenthood would be more peripheral to his daily life and therefore less costly than it would be to a woman in a similar position. Women were in fact less willing to concede the right to sterilization – for *themselves.*

Jacqueline Webster: 'I first went on the pill at 23, I wanted to be sterilized then . . . I think vasectomy would be very unfair. I mean who knows I might not be married to Andrew in five years' time. I could be killed, divorced and he marry a girl who was made to have children and change his attitude completely. A woman has an awful lot of influence over her husband in this respect because she has the child and she has the majority of the care when it's an infant and if she really loves children I don't think a man should stop her having them. And if he was sterilized he could not give her a child – he'd probably feel terrible about it and blame me.'

Women are generally more willing to consider sterilization. There is a tendency, particularly amongst more conventional husbands, to agree in principle with the abstract notion while at the same time maintaining distance between themselves and its realization.

Patricia Campbell: 'I might get sterilized . . .
Ken Campbell: 'No, I've never thought about vasectomy at all.'
Patricia Campbell: 'It'd be much easier. I don't know why I think
   it's my responsibility. I think if Ken said he'd have a
   vasectomy I'd be quite happy but as he's never brought it up
   I wouldn't like to talk him into it. You know what men are
   like . . . It's so stupid if you think about it. The woman takes
   risks taking the pill, there really is no risk with vasectomy at
   all.'

The new technology of control has allowed for this division of
responsibility which may go unchallenged where men and
women inhabit separate realities; hence the aloofness of the
more conventional male from participation in fertility control.
His rejection of vasectomy may also reflect a position he shares
with men who do not see control as an exclusively female
activity, but who nevertheless regard sterilization with a degee
of suspicion based upon popular myths linking vasectomy to
impairment or loss of virility. These prejudices are often
attributed to ignorance or lack of accurate information but beliefs
can and do persist even when contradictory evidence is recognized and acknowledged.

Douglas Johnson: 'No, I wouldn't, I wouldn't even think about it.
   I think about it but I wouldn't even ask them how much they
   were going to pay me to have it done.'
Mary Johnson: 'You might if it was for my health.'
Douglas Johnson: 'I wouldn't do it for anything . . . I'd be terrified
   of coming out with a squeaky voice. It's just prejudice.'

Other husbands favoured vasectomy – it was simpler with fewer
risks to general health.

Kate Tennant: 'I would be definitely sterilized, yes.'
Philip Tennant: 'I'm not too happy about that – sterilization is
   much more of an operation than vasectomy. It's an abdominal
   performance as far as a woman's concerned, as far as a

man's concerned, it's a couple of nicks and a couple of clips without it being an internal operation – that's it. If we were going to make a decision like that, I'd be better going for a vasectomy.'

Issues such as the relative safety of the two operations only become relevant where a couple's commitment is defined as total; even then its acceptability – as a reliable, once-and-for-all alternative to contraception – is weakened considerably by what are seen as obstacles to its availability. According to Allan Oliver: 'I'd go to-morrow if they'd take me but they won't. As far as I can make out you've got to be insane or have about three children!' This remark, although purposely exaggerated, is indicative of the frustration felt by individuals who had tried unsuccessfully to get their demand for sterilization taken seriously. Sterilization – unlike contraception – is not generally available (Allen 1981); availability is discretionary. This absence of universal criteria against which eligibility can be gauged may be one important factor behind the accusations of insensitivity and injustice levelled against the medical profession.

Jacqueline Webster: 'If a girl doesn't want a family they won't do the simplest thing like give sterilization even though the couple are prepared to sign papers and say, "It's my responsibility". If she doesn't want a family they won't sterilize her but they'll give help to people who want a family. Why not help the people who don't want a family? The doctors say, "Come back when you're 30". The majority have fobbed me off, saying, "You've only been married two years, how can you know? You're only 24, 25, 26". I first went on the pill at 23, I wanted to be sterilized then. Every so often I go to the Family Planning and the last doctor I saw was the only one sympathetic about it, who really understood that I didn't want a family. Other than that – "Oh, well you're on the pill, you're safe enough, what's your problem?". They can't understand that I'm thinking of the next 15 years I don't want to be on the pill . . . It really annoys me that you have to remember to take the pill night after night because doctors look at you and nod their heads and say, "Oh yes, I understand". As you go out the door they shake their heads, they think you're completely mad . . .

I think it's terrible that you have to rely on one person to say yes or no to you. They act as GOD.'

Even the most sympathetic of doctors, who may see childlessness as a legitimate alternative, are likely to proceed with caution in the light of the irreversibility of the operation they are being asked to perform. (Age may be used as a cautionary device: according to the reproductive timetable, the older the female, the less eligible she is, the more likely is her commitment to be total.) Total commitment, however, is not directly related to age and women in their 20s felt particularly misunderstood.

Kay Gregson: 'I think it's terribly unfair for them to say you've got to wait till you're such and such an age. It really is unfair . . . If you change your mind after you're sterilized it's hard luck . . . the gynaecologist up at the hospital said to me, "When you're older"! I said "How much older do I have to be? Give me the number of years and I'll come back and see you then". She just shrugged it off.'

Availability is a lottery apparently skewed in favour of the more articulate and the better informed – if Barbara Hargraves, working closely with the medical profession, is to be believed:

'Sterilization for me would do nothing to help the cycle and I'd be going back on the pill again so there doesn't seem to be any point in even rushing up to the local friendly neighbourhood gynaecologist and saying, "Sterilize me", which he would . . . The thing is a little bit of influence and a couple of (professional) titles . . . do help. Nobody argues with you . . . they assume you know what you're talking about.'

These impressions were substantiated by the experiences of the two couples who had obtained sterilization – in both cases vasectomy; according to Cathy McCormack, still in her early 20s:

'I've told a lot of couples it's a good idea but looking at the couples themselves they wouldn't have a hope in hell of getting it done. I think it's basically because of the people we are, we did get it done. The counselling is pretty thorough, pretty hard going and I think our attitude convinced them more than anything. I think it would be pretty hard for most couples to get it done who don't have children. You need a really sound case.'

It is unlikely that this situation has improved dramatically over the past few years. Those requesting sterilization, particularly women, are still required to undergo counselling. The childless, therefore, will continue to face the problem of finding socially acceptable justifications for what remains a decision of doubtful validity and of persuading an understandably cautious profession of the total nature of their commitment. Vasectomy appears to be more readily available (Allen 1981) and totally committed couples where the husband is prepared to take responsibility may now find sterilization a more acceptable form of control.

Commitment to childlessness obviously cannot be sustained without a parallel commitment to *preventing conception*. The childless recognize and act in accordance with this broad aim, but on the question of *preventing births once conception has occurred* there is no similar consensus. Abortion as a strategy for maintaining commitment has the childless deeply divided; some see it as the only solution to an unplanned pregnancy:

Susan Dobie: 'Now supposing by sheer accident I was pregnant, I would go automatically to the doctor and ask for an abortion that he wouldn't be prepared to give me – which I think is unfair as we're having a family forced on us that we don't want . . . Yes, I'm very much in favour of abortion. In fact I was really quite worried about it recently. My husband said, "Don't upset yourself, if the worst comes to the worst we'll take you into a private clinic or something. We'll get it somewhere".'

Others find it impossible to justify:

Rory MacDonald: 'I don't think we could consider abortion. Our feelings about not having a baby aren't strong enough to justify such an action. I think we would accept it as "destined" and react correspondingly and probably quite happily.'

And there are those who are ambivalent:

Jane Archer: 'Oh, dear, that's a difficult one. I think I'd have to face that one when it came. Oh goodness, that's really going a bit too deep. I have no idea, no. Abortion might well be an initial reaction but how far it would go, I don't know.'

Abortion is a last resort strategy, a refuge on the edge of the official culture of fertility control. On the method in principle, the childless tend to take a liberal stance – perhaps in recognition of a shared marginality – even individuals unable to give wholehearted support will neither condemn nor lightly pass judgement upon women who resort to termination. The whole issue is nevertheless fraught with moral overtones. Few couples discussed it in purely pragmatic terms; for the majority, an accidental pregnancy would involve choosing between two 'evils'. Without adequate justification the strategy would be rejected and withdrawal from commitment to childlessness inevitable. (Only one couple saw adoption as a way out of this dilemma.)

Allan Oliver: 'When it comes to abortion, I've got misgivings. I can understand it, in a lot of cases I'm all for it but if there's nothing wrong with the bairn in the womb and there's nothing wrong with the people as such – hereditary diseases or that – I feel that, okay, it's a mistake but the mistake's been made . . . If you fell pregnant and we had the opportunity to have an abortion, I don't think I would take it, then again I don't have it.'
Brenda Oliver: 'That's different, we're married . . . I wouldn't, not when you're settled.'

The Olivers were unable to justify termination: they and most other couples whose decision to remain childless had been taken to protect some aspect of the childless way of life believed abortion to be too high a price to pay for peace and quiet, a standard of living, career ambitions, a social life, and even a marriage. There were of course no couples in the study who had faced this dilemma and withdrawn commitment; one woman had however made a hypothetical withdrawal when faced with a 'false alarm'.

Joan Ellison: 'I took the first course of pills and my period didn't come and I took the second course and it was supposed to come on the Sunday and it didn't come till late on the Sunday night following and it only lasted two days and even yet I'm not convinced that I have had it. I had all that time to think maybe I was pregnant and it didn't worry me I was pregnant . . . it never crossed my mind that I would have an abortion.'

Joan Ellison enjoys her childfree life-style, is admittedly jealous of her freedoms, her marital relationship, her standard of living, but would not envisage an abortion. Carol Blair, on the other hand, having found herself in a similar situation, believed she would:

'Pregnancy does worry me, yes. In fact, it's really very amusing because recently, yes, I had a sort of false alarm, not a false alarm, but a fright thinking, "Crikey, surely not!" And I was really worried about it, you know, I was getting to the stage of thinking, well, you know, "I wonder what the chances are of an abortion?" We do both believe in abortion. And now that I'm sort of, well, coming up to 36 and I don't know what the rules and regulations about abortion are, but I think probably I'd be able to get one. But about a couple of years ago, I think, or maybe a little longer than that, say before I went to university, if I'd found I was pregnant, I think I'd have thought, "Oh well, that's it, I'll just try and do the best I can". I don't think I'd have contemplated abortion. Now I think I definitely would, I would be very, very upset if I found I was having a child, I think. About two years ago, I thought this is it and I went and had a pregnancy test and felt so relieved when I 'phoned up and found it was negative. I thought if I ever need any proof, because my immediate reaction was relief, no sort of pang of disappointment or anything.'

Carol Blair's perspective on childlessness had changed. Her initial decision had been based on a desire to protect her life-style, but the motive that had emerged and now dominated her thinking was the notion of parenthood as loss of control over self and future. She could no longer tolerate the idea of herself as mother. Others who had rejected parenthood had never visualized themselves in the parental role; they had never been committed to the values that support conventional family life and were willing to use any means available to maintain their voluntary commitment to childlessness. According to Jeannie Maxwell, who was one of two women who had had abortions, the costs of being a parent far outweigh the costs of termination.

> 'Two years ago I had an abortion, so you can tell how anti-having children I am. I'd been on the pill since '67, I came off for the most stupid reason . . . I then used the diaphragm and in a moment of drunken madness forgot to use it. It'll *never* happen again.'

A child in the picture now would totally destroy not just a way of life but an image of herself that has emerged out of conscious rejection of parenthood; it is the extent to which negative notions of the parental role feature during the early stages of commitment that tends to differentiate those who accept from those who reject abortion as a last resort strategy. Becoming a parent appears so alien as to be beyond contemplation, as this emotional statement from Susan Dobie illustrates:

> 'Supposing I had a suspicion I was pregnant and went to the doctor and he said, "Yes, you are". I'd be so terrified that I just wouldn't be able to come home because I know the effect it would have on him and that would upset me more than anything else. I just couldn't come home to face him, it would be too much for me . . . To me it would be like for someone to tell me he'd been killed in an accident. That would be the effect it would have on me.'

She had been refused sterilization.

8

Conclusion and afterthoughts

Who becomes voluntarily childless? The answer would appear to be anyone, given the 'right' situation. In other words, voluntary childlessness is not a pathological condition, but a process, the nature and purpose of which may vary as the situations out of which it emerges change. No one set of circumstances, no one social position, no one value hierarchy determines the childless response; 'the organization of a human society is the framework inside of which social action takes place and is not the determinant of that action' (Blumer 1969: 87). Describing situations does not explain action; it is necessary to grasp the way in which the situation is perceived and interpreted if the outcome – here the decision to remain childless – is to be understood.

The decision to remain childless stems from one of two basic positions. Individuals are motivated either to *avoiding the penalties of parenthood* or to *protecting the rewards of childlessness*. The positions are not mutually exclusive. Individuals, as their circumstances change and external pressures for them to conform grow, may supplement, modify, and reject as redundant their initial motivation (Veevers 1980). They nevertheless remain aware of the distinction between motives that informed and those that emerged out of their commitment to childlessness.

Avoiding the penalties of parenthood

Individuals who reject parenthood do so on the basis of their experience and observation of family life. It is with the family that socialization for parenthood begins. (Fox, Fox, and Frohardt-Lane 1982); mothers and fathers in particular, providing through their words and deeds a ready-made interpretation of family life and of the child's place within it, lay the foundations of commitment to adult roles. Commitment will not always be to the nuclear family ideal of 'two parents, 2.4 children, father breadwinning, mother housekeeping, each family in a home of its own' (Oakley 1982: 242), the epitome of cereal-packet harmony, for out of the daily round of interaction can emerge negative interpretations of the parental role: parenthood as loss of control over self and future, as a complex, arduous, and demanding task, and the child as an object of dislike. The childless are able to trace these meanings back to childhood and adolescence, spent for the most part in families which did not live up to conventional expectations; they were only children, children of empty-shell marriages, of divorced parents, and of one-parent families, they had handicapped siblings or mothers who appeared as martyrs to their role. These conditions alone do not explain the decision to remain childless. Individuals from unconventional families obviously go on to marry and have children and individuals from conventional families go on to become childless. It is possible that some parents may be more successful than others in colluding to hide their failures, disappointments, doubts, and fears and in outwardly confirming the validity of conventional values. According to Laing the family is a collusive game:

'So we are a happy family and we have no secrets
    from one another.
If we are unhappy/we have to keep it a secret.
And we are unhappy that we have to keep it a secret.
And unhappy that we *have* to keep a secret/the fact/
    that we
Have to keep it a secret
And that we *are* keeping all that secret
But since we are a happy family you can see
This difficulty does not arise.'

                  (Laing, quoted in Skolnick 1978: 85)

Impression management (Goffman 1959) may, however, prove impossible as a marriage crumbles, the pressures of single-parenthood build up, or the demands of a handicapped child overwhelm: amongst the childless there are those who remember well what they saw, heard, and felt. Others believe they simply lacked the relationships that form the groundwork for commitment to parenthood; in this category are only children and women whose mothers had played the martyr to their role or openly advocated alternative life-styles.

Situations inform the meanings that become the motives behind the wish to avoid parenthood. That wish will not always be realized. Individuals have not only to want but also to be able to avoid conformity to conventional expectations. Non-conformity implies costs, and voluntary childlessness is no exception. Most childless women, for example, believed that if they wanted to remain childless, they would have to remain single; they were acting on the assumption that parenthood is in some way natural and conforming to perceptions of themselves as unnatural and abnormal. People around them, parents and friends, expected them to marry; but at least while single – in spite of the drawbacks to this status (Cargan and Melko 1982) – they were not expected to become mothers and their identity as 'childless' went undetected (unless they came out, in which case their action would be defined as bravado, the rebellion of youth). They looked for employment that might bring financial security and independence and an acceptable standard of living and tended to distance themselves socially and geographically from their more conventionally-oriented family and friends. They wanted to marry but remained sceptical of the possibility until they met prospective partners who shared their commitment.

A like-minded partner is the support that makes voluntarily childless marriage possible. Without mutual agreement such marriages cannot exist. Finding a partner for most women provided them with a novel interpretation of their situation. Men tended not to accept prevailing imagery and to reject notions of abnormality and unnaturalness. They argued that marriage was a private affair and if they said their wives were normal and feminine, then normal and feminine they were. A minority of women, university-educated, in professional occupations, 'children of the 1960s', believing in self-determination and liberation, had developed a similar perspective and had seen no reason why they should not marry. Childless marriage was for them a legitimate alternative.

Protecting the rewards of childlessness

The desire to remain childless emerges out of stable, long-standing relationships. Individuals, previously committed to parenthood, decide to forego this option in order to maintain, foster, and protect the advantages of living together without children. Childlessness becomes comfortable routine, personal fulfilment, and marital harmony. The situations favouring the emergence of these meanings differ markedly; couples who wish to preserve a comfortable routine tend to be conventional in their life-style and interpretation of the gender roles and to become childless by default. For a variety of reasons they find themselves out of phase with the reproductive timetable; a situation which leads them to question and to perceive as superfluous the taking of what would otherwise have been an inevitable passage into parenthood; and anyway, as they themselves argue, are they not 'too old'? These are conventional couples whose nonconformity is restricted to their unwillingness to conform to reproductive expectations and who, when challenged, can excuse their actions on account of their age. Quite different, are couples who see childlessness as personal fulfilment, who tend towards androgyny, and whose decision was based on rational assessment of their situation. They have simply extended the notion of planned parenthood to include the option – no parenthood. Their decision is based on a flexible hierarchy of values. Instead of having children, they choose to pursue careers, to fulfil ambitions, to maintain a way of life, to sustain a standard of living. Parenthood is perceived as just one amongst a number of recognized and legitimate choices; life's rewards lie within the individual's personal grasp and not as an adjunct of conventional expectations. This position is shared by those who see childlessness as marital harmony and who believe parenthood would destroy what is basic to their relationships, whether this be sexuality, emotional dependence, or companionship. They reject the dominant image that sees parenthood as the source of marital harmony but otherwise tend towards the conventional. All these couples face varying degrees of censure but are able to protect themselves through their mutual support, and as with those who make a pre-marital commitment, may distance themselves socially and geographically from likely sources of pressure.

The decision to remain childless is taken within the private sphere of the family. There is, however, a public dimension to commitment. Relationships do not exist in a vacuum and the most intimate of our activities are influenced by 'the organization of human society'. Reproduction is no exception. Over the past century throughout the industrialized world a reproductive revolution has occurred; the large family of six or more has virtually disappeared and been replaced by the two-child norm. This is not a simple reflection of the availability of more effective means of birth control; motivation has changed, people not only have but want fewer children. The reasons for this dramatic reversal are complex and varied. Ariès, for example, argues for a two-stage model: in the earlier period, the major factor was the desire for better quality children; more recently, individual self-fulfilment has dominated (Ariès 1980). Both motives, according to Lesthaeghe (1983), represent an increase in individual freedom of choice. There is no doubt that individual freedom of choice has gradually infiltrated family life once so closely bound to community and wider kin group (Stone 1977; Flandrin 1979; Shorter 1975); we choose whom we marry and we marry for love, we live in nuclear units and work for ourselves, our wives and children, we divorce when our needs are not met; soon, it is argued, all notions of duty and obligation will also disappear from the reproductive sphere, and we will parent only when we believe we will gain in personal happiness and fulfilment. As yet the cultural framework, at least on the evidence of this and other studies (Polit 1978; Payne 1978; Blake 1979; Owens 1982), does not support so self-oriented a motivation. Men and women appear still to have only one legitimate option: to become parents; this is the natural and responsible course. If, on the other hand, as Kate Tennant did, a woman publicizes the fact that she does not want children because she wants to work, she may face accusations of selfishness, of being interested only in money, of not being a 'real woman'. Her husband will be similarly, though less harshly, censured. The childless are deeply offended by the way they are perceived but have no counter-argument. Whatever explanations they give, are likely to be interpreted to fit prevailing stereotypes. But unlike the stereotypes, they were neither selfish nor unnatural but were responding to situations favourable to active decision-making (Leibenstein 1981); they had been jolted out of 'inertia' by early family experiences, by being out of step with the reproductive timetable, or by having options that conflict with the demands of parenthood. These are not contingencies (Fox, Fox, and Frohardt-Lane 1982), such as war or economic slump, that may suddenly disappear leaving reproductive values and norms intact. An increasing number of individuals are going to reach adulthood not having experienced conventional family life, or, if they have, together with other disparate 'family' situations. Voluntary childlessness is likely to continue to be one response to these early experiences. Commitment based on rejection of parenthood, however, does not represent a weakening of pronatalist ideology, though it may represent a greater facility in translating desire into action, i.e. through the increasing intimacy and exclusivity of the marital relationship and the greater educational and occupational opportunities for women. It is from these changes in the position and aspirations of women that the greatest threat to the primacy of reproductive goals for the responsible and mature adult may come. Both men and women are looking for personal happiness and fulfilment in marriage and women are demanding greater control over their lives and the right to be seen as individuals and not members of a category, female, and therefore passive, unstable, materialistic, and maternal (Oakley 1982). This imagery may be proving difficult to erase but inroads are being made and it is only a short step from rejecting the universality of the feminine woman to the notion of optional motherhood.

If men and women become free to choose, why should they not choose parenthood? Parenthood meets many emotional and psychological needs (Pohlman 1969) but, some would argue, at an increasing cost, particularly for women (Bernard 1975a; Oakley 1982; Dally 1982). Small infants and children cannot meet their own needs. In the era of the housebound wife and mother, the 1950s, women were to be at the beck and call of their infants night and day, 365 days a year, for 15 years. Even though expectations may have relaxed somewhat, it is hardly surprising that women, living within the privatized unit that is the nuclear family, continue to feel weighed down and crushed by their responsibilities: responsibilities that have become even more difficult to bear given the increasing demands on women to compete in the outside world for positions of power and prestige. Motherhood has been downgraded and is in 'crisis' (Bernard 1975a; Dally 1982). This does not mean that women do not or will not want to be mothers; it may be that they will simply feel unable to take on a role that appears so costly in terms of personal fulfilment. There is, however, evidence to suggest that women will not accept this situation and that institutional arrangements will change to allow the realization of goals both within and outside the family unit. Men appear to be more willing to accept participation in caring for and raising their children and governments may find it necessary to provide child-care facilities outside the home and to develop 'part-time, drop-in child care for parents to use as they go about their business' (Skolnick 1978: 300). It is possible that if they do not women will increasingly turn to childlessness as the 'ultimate liberation' (Movius 1976).

Appendix 1

Research method

Since the aim of the study was to trace, describe, and analyse voluntarily childless careers, the most suitable research method seemed to be the unstructured, tape-recorded interview. Husband and wife were interviewed together but were allowed the possibility of private comment on the transcripts they each received for correction and amendment.

WHO WERE THE RESPONDENTS?

Participants in the research were to be voluntarily childless married couples – defined as couples in which both partners share the intention to remain childless. The stress is upon intention and agreement. This excludes from the study couples who remain childless but do so either in a state of disagreement, or unintentionally on the part of one partner unaware of the other's unilateral commitment. In neither of these cases has there been an interlocking of reproductive careers leading to the emergence of the voluntarily childless marriage. In the latter case a joint career may have emerged, but one of sterility and not of voluntary childlessness. These couples were not included. Also excluded were couples cohabiting on either a short- or long-term basis on the grounds that they again, although congruent as to reproductive intentions, inhabit a divergent social world: a divergence resulting from the numerous social and personal expectations – including many relating to parenthood –

attendant upon entering into marriage but most likely absent from the more informal type of relationship. No other criterion apart from the common-sense proviso that marriages were to have been contracted prior to the female menopause, informed the selection of couples as voluntarily childless.

Respondent profiles

Respondents were contacted at family planning clinics located in a Scottish city. Doctors monitored 'patients' who expressed the intention of remaining childless. First contact was therefore usually through the wife, who was interviewed partially to ascertain the extent to which she and her husband were in agreement over the professed commitment to childlessness. Where there was apparent disagreement the wife was not asked to co-operate. Over a 10-month period 46 primary contacts were made giving access to 92 individuals, 78 of these eventually agreeing to be interviewed. Respondents proved to be willing, eager, and able to discuss and describe their experiences articulately and in detail. They were, of course, volunteers, which is perhaps indicative of a desire and ability to com-

Table 1   Selected characteristics of the respondents

	Wives (N = 44)	Husbands (N = 34)
Socio-economic status		
I (Professional occupations etc)	7	10
II (Intermediate occupations)	19	14
III Non-manual (skilled occupations)	13	3
III Manual (skilled occupations)	1	4
Member of the Armed Forces	0	1
Full-time student	1	2
Housewife	3	0
Level of schooling attained		
Left as soon as old enough	10	6
Stayed on but no qualifications	3	0
Stayed on till 16/18 with some qualifications	16	11
College of education/art college	3	5
University/polytechnic	11	10
Mature student	1	2

municate – for many the experience appeared to offer a welcome opportunity to put their case and impart their views to what they saw as a 'sympathetic stranger'. But not only did the group consist of volunteers, it was also skewed in favour of the higher status, better-educated section of the community: a further aid to communication. Their characteristics are summarized in *Table 1*.

This concentration may be a function of the monitoring process. Higher-status women may be more willing to admit to and to discuss their childless intention. It may also reflect the unrepresentativeness of clinic attendance, but whether this tendency amongst women from Social Classes IV and V to boycott clinics includes the voluntarily childless is perhaps doubtful since the latter's motivation to avoid pregnancy might be expected to outweigh any negative attitudes they might have towards the family planning clinic. A further explanation is that the individuals contacted do in fact represent an approximation of the voluntarily childless population. There is some indirect but by no means conclusive support for this view from a national fertility survey carried out in England and Wales by Peel and Carr (1975). They found that women expressing a preference for childlessness tended to come from among the better-educated and from among those of higher status; 7 per cent of wives whose husbands were either professional or white-collar workers preferred to remain childless in comparison with 3 and 0.4 per cent among the wives of skilled and other manual workers respectively.

WHO CO-OPERATED?

Seventy-eight individuals, 44 women and 34 men representing 44 marriages, were interviewed. Where one partner failed to participate it was invariably the husband. Among those 10 who failed to co-operate three could see little point in their participation since they had all along abrogated reproductive responsibility to their wives; two, including a self-professed hater of sociologists, were not prepared to discuss their 'private affairs' with anyone; of the remaining five, two had been lost to the study after separating from their wives, the other three simply refused giving no reason. Information about all these men was gained from their wives and although not a satisfactory solution the wife's comments offered not only useful bio-graphical material but also some insight into the husband's views and experiences within the context of their shared commitment. What is missing, however, is the depth and comprehensiveness of the picture gained from descriptive accounts and from the informative discussion and repartee that took place where both partners were present.

Appendix 2

The Respondents

1 Christine Blake (20) and John Blake (23); married 2 years
2 Carol Blair (36) and Henry Blair (38); married 10 years
3 Stevie Ainsworth (26) and Peter Ainsworth (27); married 2 years
4 Jane Archer (25) and Graham Archer (26); married 4 years
5 Pauline Adams (22) and Bob Adams (26); married 3 years
6 Patricia Campbell (34) and Ken Campbell (35); married 5 years
7 Sarah Miles (32); married 4 years
8 Helen Donaldson (27) and Ian Donaldson (27); married 5 years
9 Hilary Dexter (25) and Alan Dexter (29); married 6 months
10 Susan Dobie (26); married 3 years
11 Joan Ellison (34); married 6 years
12 Mary Fraser (42); married 19 years
13 Liz Finlay (30); married 3 years
14 Kay Gregson (25) and Bill Gregson (25); married 4 years
15 Lesley Graham (25) and Andrew Graham (25); married 4 years
16 Rosemary Hall (30); married 5 years
17 Betty Hamilton (23) and John Hamilton (24); married 5 years
18 Barbara Hargraves (28) and James Hargraves (38); married 3 years
19 Sheila Kidd (27) and Donald Kidd (30); married 2 months
20 Anna Irvine (41) and Tom Irvine (50); married 10 years
21 Peggy Lawrie (42) and Reg Lawrie (43); married 14 years
22 Isobel Lomax (32) and Stuart Lomax (35); married 9 years
23 Mary Johnson (22) and Douglas Johnson (21); married 18 months
24 Ellen Kennedy (25) and Roy Kennedy (31); married 3 years
25 Ann Knight (23) and Paul Knight (24); married 4 years
26 Cathy McCormack (26) and Bob McCormack (28); married 5 years
27 Diane Marshall (28) and Graham Marshall (28); married 4 years

28 Edwina McCausland (38) and Jim McCausland (56); married 14 years
29 Claire McDonald (35) and Rory McDonald (35); married 9 years
30 Marjorie Nelson (31) and Robert Nelson (29); married 10 years
31 Sandra O'Neill (30) and Jimmy O'Neill (34); married 7 years
32 Kim Lind (26) and Paul Lind (27); married 18 months
33 Elaine Morrison (29); married 3 years
34 Brenda Oliver (23) and Allan Oliver (24); married 5 years
35 Evelyn Quin (32) and Charles Quin (33); married 3 years
36 Connie Stevenson (29) and David Stevenson (28); married 18 months
37 Maggie Smith (39); married 15 years
38 Lesley Todd (31) and Martin Todd (30); married 2 years
39 Kate Tennant (33) and Phil Tennant (37); married 10 years
40 Jeannie Maxwell (29); married 11 years
41 Carol Thompson (31); married 10 years
42 Ellen Vernon (30) and Mike Vernon (26); married 2 years
43 Jacqueline Webster (25) and Andrew Webster (28); married 2 years
44 June Young (29) and Geoff Young (27); married 2 years

References

Allen, I. (1981) *Family Planning, Sterilization and Abortion Services*. London: Policy Studies Institute.

Allport, G. (1955) *Becoming*. Princeton: Yale University Press.

Andorka, R. (1978) *Determinants of Fertility in Advanced Societies*. London: Methuen.

Ariès, P. (1980) Two Successive Motivations for Declining Birth Rates in the West. *Population and Development Review* 6(4): 645–50.

Becker, H. S. (1963) *Outsiders*. New York: The Free Press.

Berger, P. L. and Kellner, H. (1970) Marriage and the Construction of Reality. In H. P. Dreitzel (ed.) *Recent Sociology No 2*. London: Macmillan.

Berger, P. L. and Luckmann, T. (1967) *The Social Construction of Reality*. Harmondsworth: Penguin.

Bernard, J. (1975a) *The Future of Motherhood*. New York: Penguin.

—— (1975b) *Women, Wives, Mothers*. Chicago: Aldine.

Blake, J. (1968) Are Babies Consumer Durables? A Critique of the Economic Theory of Reproductive Motivation. *Population Studies* 22: 5–25.

—— (1979) Is Zero Preferred? American Attitudes towards Childlessness in the 1970s. *Journal of Marriage and the Family* 41: 245–57.

Blood, R. O. (1962) *Marriage*. New York: The Free Press.

Blumer, H. (1969) *Symbolic Interactionism*. Englewood Cliffs, N.J.: Prentice-Hall.

Bone, M. (1973) *Family Planning Services in England and Wales*. London: HMSO.

Bowlby, J. (1967) *Child Care and the Growth of Love*. London: Weidenfeld and Nicolson.

Box, B. (1981) *Deviance, Reality and Society*. London: Holt, Rinehart, and Winston.

Breen, D. (1975) *The Birth of the First Child*. London: Tavistock.

Brim, O. G. (1966) Socialization through the Life-Cycle. In O. G. Brim and S. Wheeler (eds) *Socialization after Childhood*. New York: Wiley.

Brittan, A. (1973) *Meanings and Situations*. London: Routledge & Kegan Paul.

Busfield, J. (1974) Ideologies and Reproduction. In M. P. H. Richards, *The Integration of the Child into a Social World*. Cambridge: Cambridge University Press.

Busfield, J. and Paddon, M. (1977) *Thinking About Children*. Cambridge: Cambridge University Press.

Caldwell, J. C. (1976) Toward a Restatement of Demographic Transition Theory. *Population and Development Review* 2(3/4): 321–66.

Campbell, E. (1984) Becoming Voluntarily Childless: An Exploratory Study in a Scottish City. *Social Biology* 30(3): 307–17.

Cargan, L. and Melko, M. (1982) *Singles: Myths and Realities*. Beverley Hills: Sage.

Cicourel, A. V. (1967) Fertility, Family Planning and the Social Organization of Family Life: Some Methodological Issues. *Social Issues* **XXIII**: 57–81.

—— (1974) *Theory and Method in a Study of Argentine Fertility*. New York: John Wiley.

Cohen P. (1976) Race Relations as a Sociological Issue. In G. Bowker and J. Carrier (eds) *Race and Ethnic Relations*. London: Hutchinson.

Cooper, C. L. and Davidson, M. J. (1982) *High Pressure: Working Lives of Women Managers*. London: Fontana.

Cuber, J. F. and Haroff, P. B. (1963) The More Total View: Relationships Between Men and Women of the Upper Middle Class. *Marriage and Family Living* 25: 140–45.

Dally, A. (1982) *Inventing Motherhood*. London: Burnet Books.

Deutsch, H. (1945) *The Psychology of Women: Volume II, Motherhood*. New York: Grune and Strattan.

Douglas, J. D. (1971) *Understanding Everyday Life*. London: Routledge & Kegan Paul.

Douglas, J. D. and Johnson, J. (eds) (1977) *Existential Sociology*. Cambridge: Cambridge University Press.

Dunnell, K. (1979) *Family Formation*. London: HMSO.

Farid, S. M. (1974) The Current Tempo of Fertility in England and Wales. *Medical and Population Studies* 27. London: HMSO.

Filmer, P., Phillipson, M., Silverman, D., and Walsh, D. (1972) *New Directions in Sociological Theory*. London: Collier-Macmillan.

Firestone, S. (1972) *The Dialectic of Sex*. St Albans: Paladin.

Flandrin, J. L. (1979) *Families in Former Times: Kinship, Household and Sexuality*. Cambridge: Cambridge University Press.

Fox. G. L. H., Fox, B. R., Frohardt-Lane, K. A. (1982) Fertility Socialization: The Development of Fertility Attitudes and Behaviour. In G. L. H. Fox (ed.) *The Childbearing Decision*. Beverley-Hills: Sage.

Freedman, D. S. and Thornton, A. (1982) Income and Fertility: The Elusive Relationship. *Demography* 19(1): 65–78.

Gibson, C. (1980) Childlessness and Marital Instability: A Reexamination of the Evidence. *Journal of Biosocial Science* 12: 121–32.

Glaser, B. L. and Strauss, A. S. (1971) *Status Passages and Their Properties*. Chicago: Aldine.

Goffman, E. (1959) *The Presentation of Self in Everyday Life*. Garden City: Doubleday.

—— (1961) *Encounters*. New York: Bobbs-Merrill.

—— (1968) *Asylums*. Harmondsworth: Pelican.

Gustavus, S. O. and Nam, C. B. (1970) The Formation and Stability of Ideal Family Size Among Young People. *Demography* 7: 43–51.

Hawthorn, G. (1970) *The Sociology of Fertility*. London: Collier-Macmillan.

Hollingworth, L. S. (1916) Social Devices for Impelling Women to Bear and Rear Children. *American Journal of Sociology* 22: 19–29.

Houseknecht, S. B. (1978) Voluntary Childlessness: A Social-Psychological Model. *Alternative Lifestyles* 1: 379–402.

Johnson, N. E. and Stokes, C. S. (1976) Family Size in Successive Generations: The Effects of Birth Order, Intergenerational Change in Lifestyle, and Familial Satisfaction. *Demography* 13(2): 175–87.

Kiesler, S. B. (1977) Post hoc Justifications of Family Size. *Sociometry* 40: 59–67.

Komarovsky, M. (1953) *Women in the Modern World: Their Education and Their Dilemmas*. Boston: Little Brown and Company.

Leibenstein, H. (1981) Economic Decision Theory and Fertility Behaviour. *Population and Development Review* 7(3): 381–400.

LeMasters, E. E. (1970) *Parents in Modern America*. Homewood, Illinois: Dorsey Press.

Leslie, G. R. (1979) *The Family in Social Context*, 4th edition. New York: Oxford University Press.

Lesthaeghe, R. A. (1983) A Century of Demographic and Cultural Change in Western Europe. *Population and Development Review* 9(3): 411–35.

Lyman, S. M. and Scott, M. B. A. (1968) Accounts. *American Sociological Review* 33: 46–62.

MacIntyre, S. (1977) *Single and Pregnant*. London: Croom Helm.

McKee, L. (1982) Fathers' Participation in Infant Care: A Critique. In L. McKee and M. O'Brien (eds) *The Father Figure*. London: Tavistock.

McLoughlin, J. (1984) The Case for the Conscientious Objector to Motherhood. *The Guardian*, Tuesday, 13 March: 10.

Malinowski, B. (1966) Parenthood – The Basis of Social Structure. In R. W. Roberts (ed.) *The Unwed Mother*. London: Harper & Row.

Matza, D. and Sykes, G. (1957) Techniques of Neutralization: A Theory of Delinquency. *American Sociological Review* 22: 664–70.

Mead, M. (1962) *Male and Female*. Harmondsworth: Penguin.

Mills, C. Wright (1940) Situated Actions and Vocabularies of Motive. *American Sociological Review* 5: 904–13.

Mitchell, J. (1974) *Psychoanalysis and Feminism*. London: Allen Lane.

Movius, M. (1976) Voluntary Childlessness: The Ultimate Liberation. *The Family Coordinator* 25: 57–63.

Mower, S. (1984) Pressures to be Pregnant. *The Sunday Times*, 9 December: 43.

Oakley, A. (1979) *Becoming a Mother*. Oxford: Martin Robertson.

—— (1982) *Subject Women*. London: Fontana.

Organization for Economic Cooperation and Development (OECD) (1979) *Demographic trends 1950–2000*. Paris: OECD.

Owens, D. (1982) The Desire to Father. In L. McKee and M. O'Brien (eds) *The Father Figure*. London: Tavistock.

Payne, J. (1978) Talking About Children. *Journal of Biosocial Science* 10: 367–74.

Peel, J. and Carr, G. (1975) *Contraception and Family Design: A Study of Birth Planning in Contemporary Society*. Edinburgh: Churchill Livingstone.

Plummer, K. (1975) *Sexual Stigma: An Interactionist Account*. London: Routledge & Kegan Paul.

Pohlman, E. (1969) *The Psychology of Birth Planning*. Cambridge, Mass.: Schenkman.

Polit, D. F. (1978) Stereotypes Relating to Family Size Status. *Journal of Marriage and the Family* 40: 105–14.

Rainwater, L. (1960) *And the Poor Get Children*. Chicago: Quadrangle.

—— (1965) *Family Design, Marital Sexuality, Family Size and Contraception*. Chicago: Aldine.

Rapoport, R. N., Fogarty, M. P., Rapoport, R. (1982) *Families in Britain*. London: Routledge & Kegan Paul.

Rex, J. (1978) British Sociology's Wars of Religion. *New Society* 44(814): 295–97.

Rindfuss, R. R. and Bumpass, L. R. (1976) How Old Is Too Old? Age and the Sociology of Fertility. *Family Planning Perspectives* 8: 226–30.

Rossi, A. S. (1964) Equality Between the Sexes: An Immodest Proposal. *Daedalus* Spring: 607–52.

Ryan, B. (1952) Institutional Factors in Sinhalese Fertility. *Milbank Memorial Fund Quarterly* 30: 359–81.

Ryder, N. B. (1979) The Future of American Fertility *Social Problems* **26**(3): 359–70.

Scanzoni, J. H. (1983) *Shaping To-morrow's Family: Theory and Policy for the 21st Century*. London: Sage.

Seidenberg, R. (1973) Is Anatomy Destiny? In J. Baker Miller *Psychoanalysis and Women*. Harmondsworth: Penguin.

Shorter, E. (1975) *The Making of the Modern Family*. New York: Basic Books.

Silverman, A. and Silverman, A. (1971) *The Case Against Having Children*. New York: David McKay.

Simmel, G. (1964) Characteristics of the Individual and the Dyad. In K. Wolff (ed.) *The Sociology of Georg Simmel*. New York: The Free Press.

Skolnick, A. S. (1978) *The Intimate Environment*, 2nd edition. Boston: Little Brown.

Stone, L. (1977) *The Family, Sex and Marriage in England 1500–1800*. London: Weidenfeld and Nicolson.

Strauss, A. (1970) *Mirrors and Masks: The Search for Identity*. Mill Valley, California: Sociology Press.

Sullerot, E. (1971) *Woman, Society and Change*. London: Weidenfeld and Nicolson.

Tabah, L. (1980) World Population Trends: A Stocktaking. *Population and Development Review* **6**(3): 355–89.

Udry, R. J. (1971) *The Social Context of Marriage*. New York. J. B. Lippincott.

Veevers, J. E. (1972) Factors in the Incidence of Childlessness in Canada: An Analysis of Census Data. *Social Biology* **19**: 266–74.

—— (1973) Voluntary Childlessness: A Neglected Area of Family Study. *The Family Coordinator* **22** (April): 199–205.

—— (1979) Voluntary Childlessness: A Review of Issues and Evidence. *Marriage and Family Review*: 1–70.

—— (1980) *Childless by Choice*. Toronto: Butterworths.

Waller, W. and Hill, R. (1951) *The Family: A Dynamic Interpretation*. New York: Holt and Co.

Walsh, D. (1972) Varieties of Positivism. In P. Filmer *et al. New Directions in Sociological Theory*. London: Collier-Macmillan.

Wrong, D. (1961) The Oversocialized Conception of Man in Modern Sociology. *American Sociological Review* **26**: 183–93.

Yankelovich, D. (1981) New Rules in American Life: Searching for Self-fulfilment in a World Turned Upside Down: *Psychology Today* **15** (April): 35–91.

Index